Living and Dying in a Long-Term Care Facility

Living and Dying in a Long-Term Care Facility

Notes From a Nursing Home Doctor

Gilah Silber, M.D.

2007

Living and Dying in a Long-Term Care Facility

Contents

Acknowledgment

With many thanks and great appreciation to my superb editor, Marie France, whose skill, dedication, hard work, thoughtfulness, and insights helped bring this book up to its full potential.

Dedication

To my best friend, my unrivaled supporter, and my most passionate critic, who has endured me, loved me, and encouraged my potential for more than twenty years, no matter how many times I have "dissed" you (for real and in jest). May we grow old together!

To my children, who have encouraged me to give to others as well as to our family. In return, I hope to hand over the world to you as a somewhat better place and to teach you the skills to make a difference. I promise, I will age gracefully.

To my parents who love me, let me have my own opinions, and who took good care of their elders. I hope that you will give me the opportunity to care for you as you age. To my children's paternal grandparents, who give unconditional love and devotion to their family and who endured the Holocaust.

To the facility staff members with whom I have worked over the years, your opinions have given me a unique perspective on aging. I thank you for your expertise in daily caring and for working with me to help residents with their problems. To you who have called me at three a.m., expecting to get a short answer to a problem and receiving a long, complicated one instead, I thank you for listening graciously nonetheless.

To the families of residents who act as advocates and who listen to my opinions as much as I listen to yours. To the residents whom I have taken care of over many years. You have lived through my efforts, my mistakes, and my caring. Some of you still ask about my babies (who have grown up) before telling me your problems. This book is really for you and your successors.

To the people at my favorite shops, bars, and coffee joints who have kindly listened to my nursing home stories and opinions, without giving me yours. To the musicians, writers, and artists who inspire me and give me the energy to express myself. To the spirits who guide my writing—the outlet into which I escape to make sense of my day and to find the resolve to pick up on the next. To the real "God"—who continues to make me believe, because doing the right thing does make a difference.

Gilah Silber, M.D.
January 2006

Introduction

"God Has a Risk Manager"

Aging is part of life. Growing old is as much a phase of human development as childhood and the middle years. I sometimes think of the aging process as a return to the source. Simply stated, the elder develops in reverse.

It is true that the older years are associated predominantly with loss. Losses of friends, career status, and physical functions are universal, as are losses in physical stamina and memory. Our responsibilities dwindle accordingly, to ones that require less endurance and less complex mental processing.

In the eye of the right beholder, there is an upside to this decline. Fewer responsibilities—free time—can be viewed as an opportunity to do what was not possible earlier in life. The elder gains the ability to be as carefree as a child. The ability to sleep and eat when she pleases is a benefit of aging. Some of us may even experience a sense of satisfaction in passing the baton to younger adults in the way of our possessions and even our jobs. Aging and death are ways in which we give to life.

Yet for some reason, we all look for a cure for aging, never mind that our search is akin to looking for a cure for adolescence or for toddlerhood. Why?

Some physical and emotional changes are desirable in our society; some are not. Beauty and productivity are desired (even if production leads to nothing substantial). These traits happen to be associated with the young.

Historically, elders have been esteemed sources of wisdom. Do rapid technological changes diminish the esteem in which we hold the wisdom borne of aging? Does society change so quickly now that knowledge bred from experience is defunct? Whatever the answers, it does appear that we value the traits of youth more and more, and the traits associated with age less and less. Thus part of our fear of aging is that we do not feel desirable anymore. This fear stems from a social problem, not a medical one. So why do we seek medicine to cure aging? Because science forms the basis of our beliefs and thus of our faith and hope.

As America's baby boomers age, so do their long-lived parents. As the ranks of senior citizens swell, so do the number of self-help books and expert opinions on how to deal with the "problem." My own contribution emerges out of many years as a geriatric physician. Aging, chronic illness, and death are what I deal with and think about every day. Although I have spent more than a decade caring for thousands of residents, I have not written a self-help or medical text for the layperson. Instead I like to think of my book as a "travel guide" as we embark on a demographic sea change. I intend to show how life is lived today in long-term care facilities as more of us prepare to enter them, and I offer my thoughts as to how we treat individuals at such a tenuous point in life.

Portraits of my patients point up the problems and predicaments of old age and chronic illness, some of which can be "solved" and some of which cannot. Medical issues are discussed only briefly. Individual stories speak for themselves, as do our medical, business, social, and ethical norms, which are played out in the institutions that provide long-term care.

The germ of this book arose out a visit with a patient that occurred several years ago.

Sally Ballard was the twentieth resident I would see that day on my morning rounds. I saved her for last, as she was always easy to care for, despite her many afflictions—nearly blind, hard of hearing, and ambulatory only with a walker. Steady, if slow, her mind was largely intact. She required little attention from me over the years, and I saw her only once a month. In fact, I assumed that she did not quite know who I was. That particular morning, however, she surprised me.

"I've been waiting for you," she said, and handed me a note.

I opened the folded piece of paper and read what Sally had written in a neat scrawl with a ballpoint pen.

I am an intruder, observer, spectator, bystander, and witness.
I work here but do not live here.
I am employed by the sky that "they" say is blue, yet I don't see it as blue.
The boss is purple. The clouds are green.
The boss is not God but rules us fiercer than God would—
This leader has no morals.
I know more than "you" know,
Yet I am ostracized. You have a promotion.
I am sad yet content,
I am lonely and sexy,
But I am empowered.
My wishes have been fulfilled.
I have succeeded,
But I am hopeless.
I can no longer dream.
My fears have never materialized.
I have been lucky,
But I am still afraid.
You are me but afraid of the risk.
You are managed.

I read the last line and looked up into Sally's eyes, amazed. "I had no idea that you wrote poetry," I said.

"Oh, it's nothing," she laughed.

"Not true. What you've shown me is something, really something."

Sally looked away from me, and I realized that I may have embarrassed her. Quietly I examined her and jotted down my unremarkable findings on her chart. It was time to leave. I fished into my pocket to return her poem.

"Please, keep it," she said, and gave my hand a squeeze.

Our eyes met. Spontaneously, I reached over and hugged her—something that I learned to do from patients like her.

"Thank you for letting me read what you think," I whispered into her ear.

Out in the hall, I wrote a quick note to myself: *God has a risk manager.* I would write about Sally and her poem one day.

God has a risk manager. What do I mean by that?

In Sally's poem, I read some of my own concerns as a physician in long-term care. *You are managed*, she wrote. Indeed I am. So, certainly, is she. We all are, staff and residents alike. Have we come to manage so much that we would manage (and muzzle) God, too, if we could? Is hedging against loss, misfortune, or injury—as we do in long-term care—more important than compassion and humility? What drives us to expend our energies on combating the unchangeable—meaning aging and death—yet retracting when we should reach out to comfort and to offer simple, human companionship? Does documentation shield us not only from lawsuits but also from honest acknowledgment of what it is to age and to die?

Obviously, these questions are not readily answered. They are the kind that I ask myself, though, as I drive from one long-term care facility to another. They are questions that underlie the pages of this book.

1

The Way We Age Now

Most people have known someone in a nursing home. Yet few people quite realize what day-to-day life is like there, both for the residents and for the people who take care of them—people like me.

For the past ten years, I have made the rounds as a nursing home doctor. These years have given me some appreciation of life and work in long-term care, in what appears to be a world apart. These years have given me something else as well, namely, a clear sense of how this supposed world apart connects to the world outside with respect to business, science, culture, and ethics.

In the not-too-distant past, religion formed the basis of our beliefs. Religion wove rituals all through our lives, from birth to death. Individuals took responsibility for their faults—or failed in the eyes of God. Now, many of us place our faith in science (medicine), business, and social norms as reflected in law and politics and executed by government. These systems have taken control of our lives—from birth to old age and death. Blame has shifted accordingly. Now, when things go wrong, the fault is variously ascribed to malpractice in medicine, greed in business, or to a corruption of social norms that has led to a pervasive absence of ethics. True religion, by which I mean a logical and ethical system, has been marginalized—an extracurricular pursuit for those so inclined.

Of course these shifts in emphasis have far-reaching consequences on how we cope with aging and dying. Long-term care facilities are bound to reflect the science, business, and social values that guide us overall. Such facilities are tightly regulated institutions. The rigorous government regulations that guide their every action are rooted in science and economics. Deviation from the rules is punished, both through legal fines (some substantial) and through low marks on a governmental rating system, which can have a bad effect on the bottom line.

Many people live in these facilities, not because they could not live at home, but because their presence in these institutions better accommodates and promotes the interests of business, science, and our current norms and values. The vast number of long-term care facilities that exist in the United States attest to the collective choices that we have made with regard to the systems that govern our lives. How such choices are made depends a great deal on how they are presented. Good professionals believe in what they practice, and they tend to advocate accordingly. Doctors and nurses advocate medical science. Pharmacists sell drugs. Social workers may encourage hospice care as well as long-term care in general. What is believed and practiced, however, may not be the best course of action in any given case. Other options do not get considered.

For their part, elders and their families allow themselves to be shoehorned into the "packaged" options that health care professionals offer. Faced with illness and debility, elders and their families arrive at a vulnerable crossroads in their lives. Under the circumstances, time and energy are often lacking to explore other possibilities that would allow them to customize care. So they opt for the package — say, surgery and long-term care during recovery — instead of the cobbled-together, often much more labor-intensive customization of, say, dietary and lifestyle adjustments and assisted home care.

On a massive scale, we have arrived at just such a crossroads as a society. Through instances in my own practice, I wish to show how so many systems and individuals come together to create the way that we age and die now.

The long-term care facility can be described as a family home, prison, hospital, and school dormitory all rolled into one. The stereotype of a swarm of elderly women who knit and gossip all day in front of television soap operas is more the exception than the rule. Over the last decade, I have cared not only for the aged with many chronic physical problems but also the demented, the person with AIDS, the chronically mentally ill, the accident victim, the drug addict, the prisoner who has too many physical problems to remain in jail, the Vietnam Veteran with post-traumatic stress disorder, as well as the homeless with frostbite and an infected leg. There is no such thing as a typical long-term care resident.

Perhaps there is no such thing as a typical geriatrician, either. In my case, I was not born to the calling but evolved toward the profession gradually. The field of geriatrics is an intriguing mix of medicine and psychiatry. At the time that I was a student in the early 1980s, the philosophy of geriatrics was akin to mine—do no harm, help when able, and guide the resident and family in the decision-making process. I also happen to like old people. I treat their medical problems, yes. But I like to talk to them, to look at their photo albums. I like to get to know their families (even if they are sometimes belligerent).

Over time, I have come to focus on a second group within my larger practice, that is, on younger residents with chronic disease. With their complicated medical and psychiatric scenarios, these young people tend to need all the help that I can offer. Too often, they are the outcasts in the LTC facility. Interestingly, this type of resident tends to seek me out as well. Like gossip, reputations travel fast in the small, self-contained community of a nursing home. Affinity also plays its part. We size one another up and can tell when we are well suited. Work is more enjoyable if the client chooses you. In that respect, my job is no different than any other.

In the chapters ahead, I rely on composites of the residents that I have cared for. I do the same regarding the long-term care facilities and their staff. Despite their altered form, these "people" and "places" embody a large part of my life. I am eager to introduce them to you. Old age and illness are hardly static, and so we will see how these clients of mine move through predicament and ordeal, and how their changing conditions are perceived and managed by the facilities in which they live.

How immense is my responsibility and how dramatic my role, and yet how fleeting I often appear in the lives of the people I serve. Certainly my job has never been glamorous. Over the last few years, however, I have seen my role grow more bureaucratic than ever. I chose geriatrics out of a genuine desire to care for the elderly. Yet it is a rare day that I spend simply caring.

If I want to work in a nursing home, I must cater to the needs of the nursing home care team. As a consultant, I must please my clients (who extend beyond the residents themselves to their families and to the nursing home staff and administrators). I must document compliance with laws, regulations, and care plans sometimes against my better judgment, sometimes even in opposition to scientific fact. I must serve state regulators, pharmaceutical companies, and I must prove to insurance companies that they are paying for effective services. I must document my residents constantly—their weight loss, falls, and all the other natural consequences of aging. I must document death.

On-the-job incentives to simplify or minimize medical treatment are limited. In fact, the incentives are just the opposite. I am paid only for direct patient care and for what in the insurance business is called the "complexity" of medical decision making. That means that I am paid to order tests, medications, and to make changes in individual care plans. If a resident needs no test or medication, or desires none, I am paid less. If I believe that a test is not warranted to diagnose terminal cancer in a 102 year old, I will not be compensated to the same degree that I would be, had I made the "complex" decision to order the test.

As for consultative care, I am offered no monetary incentive to talk with family members, either in person or by phone. Yet I must document talks that do occur as part of long-term care management. I could be compensated for my talks with residents themselves, were I willing to document our conversations at length. For the most part, however, I am not willing. I would feel I had breached the patient-physician relationship. Despite the lack of remuneration, one of the most rewarding parts of my job is to talk over the care of residents with their families and occasionally to mediate misunderstandings about what the care team and administration are doing. This role as liaison can be quite satisfying as long as the care team has the residents' interests in mind.

Pleasing my clients, more often than not, means accepting a facility's management system and creating a good care plan. On occasion, I am forced to agree to a corporate care plan and to take the legal consequences. A mistake need not even occur. A person (usually a family member) may simply be dissatisfied and file suit to dispute the care plan in court. The precariousness of my position is not one that many physicians are willing to accept. Nor, for that matter, are many doctors drawn to aging and death, with none of the cures that they trained so long and hard to provide.

Though not wealthy, I am fairly well compensated. Still, extensive training means that I did not start to make a living until I was in my mid-thirties. All in all, I have had fifteen years of formal schooling after high school. I received an undergraduate degree in science and went through several years of graduate training before I went to medical school. I did my residency in internal medicine for three years, after which I trained for an additional two years as a fellow in geriatrics. Even as a highly educated fellow in training (at age thirty-five), I made less money than a nurse—and nurses are not well-compensated for what they do.

Despite all our efforts and training, those of us who work in geriatrics are seen, by and large, as "inferiors" in the health care community. Among our peers in the health care field are some who think we in geriatrics must be incompetent to work in any other field of medicine. Why else would we take care of old, dying people? If we were truly any good, we would have studied to become plastic surgeons, highly paid to give young women larger breasts.

At the root of the stigma lies fear—of getting old and dying. To hide our fear from ourselves, we disdain our elders as well as those who care for them. Low morale and high job turnover have a number of causes of course. Lack of professional prestige is undoubtedly among them.

For staff dealing with direct patient care, such as bathing and toileting, long-term care is not a pleasant job, on the whole. If it were, the number of people working in the field would be far higher than it is. Most professionals who do persevere do so because they have a true sense of caring for the elderly. We are not taking care of elders because we are unable to care for anyone else or did not get a residency in plastic surgery. As a matter of fact, I love my job. Perhaps this book will explain why.

This book is not meant to be negative. I do not wish to expose the long-term care facility as a bad place. I do not condemn families who cannot take care of elders or family members who are severely disabled or ill. I do not want to prove that young people who reside in a long-term care facility are lazy or irresponsible. What I do hope is to give a relatively impartial account of residents and their lives.

At home in the evenings, I often unwind at my writing desk. To jot down my thoughts and feelings leads the way out of frustration and occasionally to the solution to a problem. This book grew out of such notes written at the end of some very long days.

2

Making the Rounds

The relationship between the physician and the long-term care resident is, on the surface, not that complex. Once a resident has decided on me as a physician, I am to take care of his or her health to the best of my ability and to act on his or her behalf. Initially, I do an extensive assessment. Subsequently and by law, I see each of my patient-residents at least monthly to assess their health and well-being. Of course I see them more often if a new health problem arises or if a current one grows worse.

When residents are not too ill, I use my time to get to know them. Even in the early stages of dementia, many people, I find, still offer insights, as they regain the innocence of a child and, for a little while longer, retain access to the experience of an adult. With nothing to lose, such patients may tell me about the world as they see it, without fear for their jobs, their friendships, or their social status.

Of course, I cannot afford to be unguarded myself as I adhere to clinical guidelines, pharmaceutical guidelines, and long-term care guidelines. As a physician and the facility's medical director, I must by law:

- Provide for the medical and social needs of the residents
- Protect resident rights
- Make sure that patient-care policies are carried out
- Monitor the attending physicians
- Attend to the education of staff
- Act as liaison among family members, facility administrators, state regulators, and other relevant parties.

Not only is this description of duties a bit vague, it is also nearly unattainable. It may also be contradictory in its implications—unless we assume that the staff are interested solely in the residents and are not concerned with their own problems, which may include finance and marketing challenges, as well as internal conflicts.

If all goes well, the care I provide pleases not only the resident but the resident's family, the nursing home administration, the facility care team, the pharmacy, the insurance company, and state surveyors. Not surprisingly, pleasing all of the people all of the time rarely happens.

&

My first stop today is the Apple Lane Nursing Facility, about thirty minutes from my house. This morning I plan to see three new residents there and one of my current clients who is acutely ill. My visits come as the month of March draws to a close. By now, I have completed my routine, monthly visits to the other sixty residents whom I care for at Apple Lane.

The facility is not in a good neighborhood. As I drive toward my destination, I receive and return calls from two different facilities. It is half past six, and I will remain on call until the office of my medical practice group opens at eight. Meanwhile in my old but expensive SUV, I pass police cars that stand idle, double-parked in front of a residence, their lights flashing against the first gray light of day. A mile later, I pass another police car parked in the street. This time a few teenagers and younger children huddle nearby.

As I reach Apple Lane, I receive another call. The administrator at Fern Oakes is upset. A resident who sent herself to the ER last night has returned. Still drunk, she can be heard complaining loudly about the facility. "Can't you admit her to the hospital for something?" the administrator practically pleads. "She needs to be out of the facility while the surveyors are here."

"I'm sorry, I can't do that," I tell him, as I pull into the parking lot. (The security guards recognize my vehicle and wave me through, so I escape interrogation.) "Why not get someone to sit with her quietly for a while?" I suggest, but the administrator hangs up, dissatisfied.

I answer one more call as I get out of my car. A resident needs an order for a diet change, something easy to fix. As I cross the parking lot, there is much activity. The night shift is leaving, and the new shift is coming on duty. Several taxis pull up and depart, ferrying staff to and fro. Outside the double-glass entrance, members of the night staff smoke and talk as they wait for their rides. To the right of the building, a small grove of trees and bushes leads to an apartment project. Someone was murdered in these woods several months ago—a drug-related crime, apparently. The victim was the grandson of someone on staff, part of the core group that has been here for many years.

This core group stands in marked contrast to most of the staff. Especially at entry levels, they do not stay here long.

Transience is common. Most facilities are relatively the same, yet the people who work in them move from one to another to escape difficult interpersonal relations and endemic institutional problems. Burnout is a big problem in long-term care. Staff address the most basic human needs and witness the most intense and difficult parts of life. We are to act as professionals, but at times our own feelings are overwhelming, often compounded by conflicting requests. We deal, say, with the needs of a dying woman, while the administrator wants to cut the costs of her care and her son wonders when Mom will walk again.

Some staff leave by choice; others are asked to go. In any case, little effort is expended to keep them. Perhaps it is simply easier to replace people than to fix a situation. As it is, many members of these so-called "professional families" often lack experience and training in the roles that they are expected to fill.

At the other end of the spectrum, staff at the upper levels—administrators, admissions personnel, directors of nursing—may not recognize the residents by face but only by name, or as numbers in a field of data that make up statistics related to the facility's business profile. Day-to-day relationships with the residents are relegated to the lower ranks, whose methods are usually poorly understood by the "higher powers."

Quality assurance requires staff to consider such things as a resident's lab values, the number of days that he or she has spent in the hospital, as well as his or her pharmacy bills. What is not required is for staff to know each resident when they see them.

In the many team and quality assurance meetings that I have sat in at long-term care facilities over the years, it has not been unusual for resident care to go unmentioned.

Census data, billing, and staffing are much more likely to be discussed. It would be entirely possible to work in a long-term care facility and never realize that caring for the residents was supposed to be the goal.

❧

I enter the Apple Lane facility and am about to begin my rounds when Margo, a nursing assistant that I have known for some time, motions me over to talk privately.

"I think I have a bladder infection," she confides.

In the staff lounge, I diagnose Margo and give her an antibiotic. As I leave the lounge, I bump into another staff member, Lacey, who tells me that her grandson is ill and was in the hospital over the weekend.

"What do you think is wrong with him?" she asks me.

"I don't want to guess," I tell her.

She changes the subject. "You won't mind refilling my prescription for migraines, will you?"

"Of course not."

I go upstairs to see two new residents. A nurse at the front desk eyes me suspiciously. I have not seen her before. Luckily, Jody, a nurse who has been at Apple Lane for more than a year, gives me a smile and a wave. Everything is "kosher" now. The new nurse turns her attention away from me.

I go in to see Joe Scott. Though a new patient for me at Apple Lane, I used to see him regularly at Marwood, another long-term care facility. At fifty-five, Joe has diabetes, hypertension, and peripheral vascular disease. The last time that I saw him, he had a wound on his foot from frostbite and gangrene, the results of hypothermia after living out on the street during very cold weather. He left Marwood at the request of the administrator, who accused him of selling cocaine on the premises. Though I lost track of him after that, it is clear that he has not done well since. For one thing, he developed a severe infection and required below-the-knee amputation of his left leg.

Despite everything, Joe remains handsome—and charming. Today he looks glad to see me, as he flashes the business card that I gave him long ago. He acts as if it were remarkable for him to have one, which, under the circumstances, it is.

"If I didn't see you today," he says, "I was going to call you." His voice is the same, low and rich in tone.

Joe talks about the loss of his limb and how depressed he feels. He does not want an antidepressant, though. He wants to deal with his loss all by himself. He asks me to go over his medications with him, which I do. He would like a mild anxiolytic and a sleeping pill for a short time. The facility is noisy, and he is having trouble getting used to the din. We discuss his pain medications. He certainly has reason for pain and cause for treatment, but he is also a known drug addict and drug dealer. We come up with a pain management program that we can agree on.

"See you in a week or so," I say.

I move on to see Gloria Brandenberg. She is a new resident, not only to me but to the facility. Gloria is sixty-seven and heavy-set. Unlike Joe, she makes no effort to charm me or to disguise what appears to be a profound weariness. She has just been through a long hospitalization after a colostomy due to an ischemic bowel. Her hospitalization was complicated by respiratory distress and a wound infection. As I interview and examine her, she does not remove her pair of pitch-black sunglasses.

"I hope to get stronger with therapy," she tells me. Her voice is gravelly. "I want to have the colostomy reversed."

"That may be possible in four months or so," I say.

She grunts. "I used to be a teacher. My home was sold while I was in the hospital."

She gives me no details. I never do see her eyes.

On my way out, I take the opportunity to return a call from another facility. A resident is not eating. I ask a few questions and give a few orders.

Next I visit long-time resident Jacob Ashley, who is very ill at the moment. At forty-seven, Jacob has AIDS. I have taken care of him for nearly ten years. I also take care of his partner, who happens to be the same age as my own partner. Jacob remembers the birth of my youngest daughter (now eight) and continues to ask about her. He even remembers her name (Avishav—not too easy).

I enter his room quietly. Jacob is a night owl and usually is not up before noon. This morning, however, he is awake, awaiting my visit.

I evaluate him. He has the most beautiful blue eyes. He also has a fever and an ear infection, which I can treat simply. I tell him that I have recently seen his partner, who is doing well (in another facility). He gives me a smile as I leave him. I always wonder when I will see him for the last time.

In the hallway, I take the last call on my Sunday-to-Monday shift. The son of one of my colleague's patients wants to speak about his father. I tell him to call back in five minutes when the office will open to reach his primary physician.

I press on to pay my last visit at Apple Lane. Bruce Maynard is a new resident at the facility, who is just out of the hospital after suffering a bout of seizures. At sixty, Mr. Maynard has a history of alcohol abuse and chronic mental illness. He has no family other than a brother. At some point in his life, he used to be a social worker, he says. When he first arrived here for rehabilitation and medication management, he was placed in a regular unit but began to pick fights and harass the elderly residents. The staff then moved him to the behavioral unit, set aside for psychiatric patients, which is where I introduce myself.

"Did my lawyer, Mr. Prince, tell you to come see me?"

"No," I say.

My answer seems to puzzle him.

I must look puzzled myself.

I head back downstairs, where I wave to Pam Evans, the director of medical records and a long-time friend at Apple Lane. She invites me to her office for coffee. Pam is about my age, that is, in her late forties. Today she is anxious about her daughter, Alicia.

"Her husband beat her up real bad," she tells me. Though he is now in jail, Pam is worried. Her daughter will need time to recover. "So who's going to take care of her three kids?"

I offer what comfort I can. Then I throw my coat over my shoulders and head out to the parking lot. It is not yet nine o'clock.

3

Private Life in a Public Place

The long-term care facility, also called a nursing home, is a place for those who cannot care for their daily needs. All of these individuals live under one roof. What do they have in common? First, they have no appropriate caregivers at home, though that is where most would like to be. I have rarely met a resident who wants to spend his or her last years in a nursing home. I have, however, met people who have become satisfied with their lives in such places.

Residents also have in common a payer source—someone who is willing to pay the nursing facility for their care. The residents themselves or their families pay, insurance pays, or the state pays (for those who have no assets), for a room, meals, and round-the-clock care for basic needs, including nursing care. In an ideal world, everyone would have enough resources to support their basic needs. They would have insurance for crisis care or to cover the unexpected. They would not abuse the system if they did not need the coverage.

At the time that I write, the minimum cost of care in an American nursing home is about six thousand dollars a month. The price of room and board runs upward of one hundred and thirty dollars a night. The remaining two thousand or so dollars per month pay for a care plan, which the staff creates and carries out. The remainder also pays for a nurse or an aide to administer medications and to provide very basic hands-on care. Medications, therapy, physician visits, and diagnostic testing are not included in this amount; they are added costs. Thus: (room and board) + (nursing and other staff) + (care plan) = cost of LTC.

Let us assume that government regulations to monitor the standard of care continue to rise. Let us also assume that the monthly cost of long-term care remains the same (or increases at a slower rate than do regulatory costs). Hands-on care and the quality of the room and of the food will still decline. Quality care will probably always cost more than a profitable business can bear.

No Place Like Home

Although it may sound trivial, where we live tends to matter to most of us. We have all been to other people's homes. We have been to hotels. In few cases does the physical environment seem "right"— like home, that is. Yet people who come to live in long-term care facilities still hope to live in the way that they always have. Their desire, sad to say, is largely unrealistic.

Many LTC residents do not have a private room, which may be the result of deliberate facility design, or it may be because they cannot afford one. It may even be by choice (some people do not want to be alone). Still, the prospect of a roommate is novel for most people entering long-term care. Even those who have shared a room at college or summer camp did so at a time in their lives when they were free to come and go at will.

Think of the situation. A person leaves his home, his possessions, and his independence, often quite abruptly. In many cases, he, or his family, will have made the decision (to be placed in the LTC facility) right after an acute hospitalization or illness. He moves to what is likely to be his final living space and sleeps in a twin-sized bed next to someone (usually less than ten feet away) whom he does not know. Into a space whose dimensions are smaller than a hotel room's, the new resident will be able to bring only a few of his personal belongings, perhaps a chair and a dresser. Even if he does have a private room, he may not have a private bath.

Private life is no longer screened from public view. Personal tics and habits that have gone unnoticed by all but the closest of friends and family over a lifetime now undergo scrutiny by perfect strangers. Dining areas are communal, as are most activities. Together residents play bingo, watch movies, do crafts, attend religious services, and travel to offsite cultural events. Along the way, friends and acquaintances are made, though the pool of people with whom residents can bond is limited; usually no more than a hundred people.

Paradoxically, a person's individuality dims even as it undergoes more scrutiny than ever before. No longer able to care for themselves, for many a loss of personal identity follows on a loss of autonomy. Residents don armbands and wear identification labels on their clothing. As caregivers devise plans for their care, residents become known to them more on paper than in person. On the broadest scale, behavioral norms are standardized by government regulation. Within any given setting, however, they are also set in accordance with the values and personal opinions of the staff and administration. What is acceptable behavior in one nursing home, say, sexual activity, may not be tolerated in another.

As I recall the many facilities in which I have worked over the last decade, I could not recommend one as a place that I would choose to stay. Even the best facilities are still a long way from providing the amenities to be found in an average hotel. Even LTC residents who pay top dollar do not enjoy thick towels and soft linens, and certainly not the other perks we associate with pleasant accommodations. The food is, of course, institutional style.

Like the members of my family, I doubt that you and yours would be eager to stay at a hotel where you would share a shower and toilet with a stranger, sleep in a narrow, hard-mattressed bed, and eat food of a school cafeteria quality. And, of course, if you wanted a telephone or TV, you would have to arrange for them yourselves. Maid service could not be counted on, either, as it would depend on the availability of adequate staffing. Tipping, at least, would not be required.

Obviously, a stay at a long-term care facility differs dramatically from one in a hotel. Among other things, residents pay for a nurse to give them medicines, assess their health status, and assist them with basic needs, such as bathing. Not so obviously, the cost differential between a hotel and a nursing home does not account entirely for the lack of amenities in LTC living accommodations. In part at least, the difference reflects our social expectations of how our oldest and weakest members should live. Is a bedsheet with a high-thread count wasted on a woman with dementia? Even in cases where advanced dementia has set in and the resident is "scientifically" unaware of her surroundings, personal space can remain important—not least to her caregivers.

A Room of Her Own

My former patient Betty Chang, for example, was unable to help move her own body. Her aides needed to use what is called a "Hoyer lift" to give her the extensive care she needed throughout the day. A tiny room or a shared room would have made more arduous the job of changing this incontinent woman several times a day.

Oblivious to the room's décor, Betty did smile at the sight of the framed family photos at her bedside. There was not much left to her life otherwise, except being changed, being bathed, and having her family visit her. She did not care what the food was like, as she did not eat. Her one remaining pleasure of the senses seemed to be listening to the radio, and she would tap her foot to Benny Goodman and sway to the sound of a waltz. A private room meant that Betty could listen to music all day long without bothering another soul. Interestingly, that room did not turn out to be her final home, as explained later in this chapter.

Wide Open Spaces

Entirely different kinds of patients also may benefit from a change in physical space. Justin Williamson could not have cared less about his surroundings when he first came to live at the long-term care facility. No wonder. He could not maneuver much in any case, weighing more than five hundred pounds. All of his physical problems stemmed directly from his obesity, but they were significant—diabetes and hypertension, severe osteoarthritis (which means that he was unable to walk), and congestive heart failure (which caused massive swelling in his lower extremities). This swelling caused weeping of fluid from his skin and open sores to develop. Though he was but thirty-eight years of age, he could not ambulate, transfer, or bathe himself. His anatomy was so contorted that he could not urinate on his own.

Before his arrival at the facility, he had lived in an old house in a poor neighborhood. There, he could not go up the steep stairs or even move from room to room without significant effort, given the cramped entryways and narrow halls. He relied on others to manage his personal space as well as his bodily functions and to position his wheelchair where he could view the television set, his main source of contact with the outside world. In fact, it was his confinement that had led to his transfer into long-term care in the first place. He had developed skin wounds and was hospitalized for sepsis. During his hospitalization, it became clear that he required more intensive medical care than his family could give him at home.

Within a short time of his arrival at the facility, Justin's life began to change. His own private room still held little meaning, as he remained unable to maneuver in a small environment. What made a difference were the communal areas. The modern facility was accessible, even for a bariatric (obese) resident as large as he was. There was a wide elevator that he could manage alone, and the doorways and the hallways were also large enough to accommodate him and his electric wheelchair. New independence led to a new life, one in which he could plan each day and make choices.

Justin chose to wheel himself to physical and occupational therapy, and he started learning how to do special exercises in line with his physical condition. He participated in social activities, where he made some friends. With easy access to and from the facility, he was able for the first time in many years to get outside on his own and wheel himself down to the corner store.

Also different from home were the controlled meals. Not only were the ingredients regulated, but his old habit of crying for what he wanted did not have the same effect on the staff that it did on his mother and sister. The facility gave him a greater opportunity than he had ever had before to change his life and improve his health, if he chose.

Outlook and Adjustment

Most of the people who live in such facilities are elderly but—as we just saw at Apple Lane—some are chronically mentally ill with medical problems, and they include the middle-aged. Even quite young persons, such as Justin Williamson, can be found in long-term care, albeit with debilitating physical problems. Though it is a generalization, age and experience do affect how well residents adjust to life in long-term care.

The Older Resident

Typically, the older person is whom we expect to find in long-term care. Yet the life of such a person is often too complex to be called typical, given the varied expectations after a lifetime rich in experience. Cognitively intact residents bring their memories with them. Most likely, they have raised a family and held a job. They have run a household and amassed material goods. Over the years, they may have mastered a few talents and cherished hobbies. Some have had a chance to travel. Not surprisingly then, lucid elders are the residents most likely to be dissatisfied with the long-term care experience, which can underscore all that they once had but now have lost.

Mentally deficient residents, on the other hand, may be content with the same environment precisely because they have a dim or confused recollection of the lives they once led and because they are not fully aware of their present surroundings. Still, even the mentally deficient may express dissatisfaction through regression and other dysfunctional behavior. My former patient Gilbert Pollick comes to mind. His history of chronic mental illness, particularly paranoia, complicated his old age and made it quite difficult for him to adjust to life in a nursing home.

The Younger Resident

Adapting to life in long-term care can be easier for young people than it is for elders, given their relative lack of experience and limited opportunities elsewhere. Ease in adaptation occurs especially among young people whose reasons for entering into long-term care are genetically based. A disease like multiple sclerosis or diabetes makes infirmity an integral part of life, as do other conditions that are chronic. Such a resident is more likely than most to be satisfied with the long-term care experience and to accept the facility as home. That was certainly true of Justin and his friends.

In recent years, long-term facilities have begun to see a rise in bariatric patients like Justin, that is, the morbidly obese. In fact, Justin was not alone among such patients that I cared for at his facility. Two other residents were nearly as obese as he was. The three of them became fast friends and adapted quickly to life in the facility. Together they ordered food out, smoked cigarettes, and watched television side by side in their wheelchairs.

Angry Young Newcomer

On the other hand, a resident whose disability stems from an accident is more likely to be bitter, angry, and careless. That was true of Greg Farmer, who came to live in a nursing facility when he was twenty-nine, paralyzed from the neck down after a drunken dive into an empty swimming pool. Greg represented another kind of newcomer to long-term care, one who would not have lived without the intervention of modern medicine. As recently as twenty years ago, he would have died from the injuries that he sustained. Instead, specialized trauma care and extensive therapy enabled him to survive, although not without round-the-clock care and not without emotional misery.

Greg came to long-term care mean and angry. He took his unhappiness out on the staff, calling them "sluts," "whores," and "bitches." Just as he abused his caregivers, he misused his medical care. To keep some sense of autonomy, he kept making random and contradictory decisions about his care, refusing to cooperate one month and demanding new medications the next. He never did adapt so much as he circled viciously. His abuse was self-destructive and led to further reliance on cutting-edge technology, leading to multiple hospitalizations and surgeries including a colostomy. Each time he returned to the facility in a poorer condition than when he left. His mind, however, continued to be clear.

The Acts of Living

Each resident spends a great deal of time on ADLs (activities of daily living)—toileting, dressing, bathing, ambulating, and eating. These essentials of life may be performed independently, with some assistance, or with total dependence on caregivers. Given the limitations of staffing, dependent residents may receive help from three different people daily. The situation is akin to a newborn having three different mothers, each with her own habits and expectations. Staff transience also hurts residents in this regard. The elderly or chronically ill person, who needs security and familiar faces, instead is greeted by a series of strangers. The people behind the faces, to reiterate, may well suffer from low morale and high stress on the job. These silent factors directly affect the care of the resident. If relationships are short-lived, they can be powerful. The window of opportunity for staff to make a positive difference is small. Unfortunately, so is the time to make up for a mistake, such as handling an elder roughly while giving him a bath.

Some residents are able to perform a few instrumental activities of daily living (IADLs), which require more advanced functions— handling finances, preparing meals, shopping, traveling, and performing housework. Other common activities include visiting family members, engaging in hobbies, reading, attending facility events, and participating in scheduled outings. Activity and social interaction are important enough to lead regulators to penalize facilities that offer too few planned functions for their residents. Staff have no ability, on the other hand, to regulate how residents respond. They cannot force them to join in—let alone enjoy—such activities.

The Color of the Bigger Picture

Beyond the hours of the day lie a multitude of belief systems based in science, business, social norms, and ethics. These systems and values color life in long-term care, just as they do life elsewhere in twenty-first-century America. The proliferation in long-term care facilities itself reflects a shift in social controls. Whereas in the not too distant past, religion dominated the life cycle and ritualized every pivotal event, including death, the last-quarter century has witnessed a takeover in control by medicine, politics, and business. As we have already seen, advances in medicine have increased the number of residents in long-term care. A few decades ago, the dialysis patient, the paraplegic, the stroke victim, and the person on a feeding tube would have died, making long-term care a moot point. Today's survivors require care that is often too difficult and strenuous for their families to perform. To receive the medical care that they need to remain alive, they must enter intensive care at a long-term care facility.

Yet there are other reasons for the rise in long-term care, too. Making money is certainly one of them. Keeping people in long-term care provides a steady income to various enterprises and professions. Sending residents home does not. Though it is true that some people could not live anywhere else, others could do just as well with home-based assistance. Such turned out to be the case for Betty Chang, one of my first patients after I finished my fellowship.

Going Home

Betty had always appeared to be an ideal candidate for long-term care. At eighty-three she had multiinfarct dementia, the result of a series of strokes, and her mental status was extremely compromised. In many ways like an infant, she was unable to feed herself, toilet herself, walk, or speak. Minimally responsive to caregivers and family members alike, she seemed perfectly content to spend her last days listening to music on the radio in her private room in the nursing facility.

It came as a surprise when her daughter, Susie, decided to take Betty home. The facility was opposed to the idea, and I also was reluctant to let her go. In the end, however, I authorized home care and persuaded my colleagues to let her daughter give it a try. Susie's days would consist of feeding, changing, bathing, and giving her mother medications. We all assumed that Betty would be back in permanent long-term placement in short order. We were wrong.

From the outset, the Chang family thought ahead. At their request, I continued to serve as Betty's physician, given Susie's remote location, where quick access to another physician would be only by way of an ambulance. The Changs likewise arranged for weekly respite care from a series of home health aides and nurses so that Susie could get a break. She herself called me frequently with questions, and sometimes I prescribed medications.

Nonetheless, Susie had her own ways to care for her mother. She would not let her gain weight, as she would then not be able to lift her. She used foods other than the standard formula in her tube feedings. Occasionally, she took Betty off her tube altogether for a few days and substituted juices, a long-term care "crime." When she was a child, Susie had had cancer. She attributed her survival to her mother's care. Susie wanted to offer the same care to her mother, which included the juice fast.

Eight years later, Betty was still at home. She never had a bedsore or any major problem. Susie knew her mom and knew how to take care of her.

Ironically, the only mishaps occurred during the two or three times a year when Betty re-entered long-term care while Susie took a vacation. Once both her legs were broken in a transfer from the bed to the bath. Several times, she developed bedsores. None of these facilities was a bad place or negligent in its care. Such things do happen even with the best of care. "There is no place like home."

All Business

Few things can be done for the elderly or the chronically ill in a long-term care facility that cannot be done for them at home. That being said, many of us, for many reasons, are simply not prepared to care for our elderly parents around the clock. In my town I can recall a lawyer who went to a great deal of trouble and expense to care for her aged parents, who needed twenty-four-hour supervision plus nursing care.

Lisa Cox, and her husband built an "elder-friendly" addition onto their house so innovative that it was featured in a local magazine spread. This woman was equally adept at arranging and hiring quality care for her parents. She had a plan, and a back-up plan, for caregivers. She arranged through a service for physicians to make house calls so that her parents need not wait in long lines for medical care. Hot meals and a twenty-four-hour sitter service were in place. All was well, until one night when the primary caregiver was unavailable, and the back-up caregiver did not answer her phone. All of a sudden, Lisa was unable to cope. She barely made it through twelve hours alone with Mom and Dad and soon opted to put them into long-term care.

That she opted for the business model to care for her parents came as no surprise. Throughout her entire adult life, Lisa had been relying on business transactions to provide her family with care at every stage. First she birthed her children according to her obstetrician's advice. Then she raised her babies according to what her pediatrician told her was right, as well as by reading the latest books by the current leading experts on infancy. Once her children reached toddlerhood, she put them in day care, and later when they entered school, they took on a plethora of after-school activities that continued from that point on until they went away to college. Their home, meanwhile, was merely a place to stop by in between "activities," just as it was a way station for Lisa and her husband to stop by between "appointments."

Eventually, the couple's children married and had children of their own. Lisa loved her grandchildren and spoiled them (but did not take care of them). As she was fond of saying, Lisa enjoyed her "own" life. By choosing the business model, she could hide from herself as well as her family the inability to nurture and care for another human being. If her inability was due in part to inexperience, the business model helped perpetuate the lack.

Her parents lived long lives. Lisa's mother was ninety-eight before she entered my care and was diagnosed with metastatic adenocarcinoma of unknown origin, a grave diagnosis and virtually incurable. Given the gravity of the diagnosis and her mother's advanced age, it was easy to assume that Lisa would opt for hospice care. This time, however, Lisa surprised me. One of her clients was an oncologist and a leading expert in the field. After consulting with him extensively, Lisa decided on aggressive diagnostic tests and treatment. For the next two weeks, she took time away from her legal practice to spend her days arranging diagnostic tests, visiting specialists, and searching the Internet for cures and treatments for this fairly rare and deadly disease. She called me frequently, updating me on the progress of her pursuit. Her visits to her mother consisted of chauffeuring her to and from specialists. As for her dad, she had no time to visit him at all during this period.

Several weeks after her diagnosis, Lisa's mom entered the hospital for intensive chemotherapy and radiation. On the same day, Lisa's dad fell at the long-term care facility and broke his hip. A few days later, Lisa's mom passed away. She had undergone only one treatment of radiation, which she was not strong enough to withstand. Lisa's dad, meanwhile, underwent surgery on his hip, unaware that his wife had died.

The funeral and burial were preplanned affairs, executed with swift precision. No sooner were they over than Lisa returned to her computer to search the Internet, this time for new cures for her dad's osteoarthritis, osteoporosis, and hip fracture. She hired a therapist and a specialist as part of her effort to find a cure for what ailed her aged father.

Once again, Lisa sidestepped personal and affectionate care. Clearly she could not bear to stand by her dying parents. First she used the business model and hired people to take her place and thus keep anxiety and pain at arm's length. Later she relied on the scientific model and lost herself in tireless bouts of research and rounds of tests. In each case, she buried her anguish in the face of a hopeless cause. First one parent died and then the other. Rationality and efficiency were what she knew; natural grieving and caring were not.

If we cannot care for our elders and our chronically ill relatives at home, we can buy a "plan" that will deal with them for us. In turn, we forfeit some of our autonomy as a family. Not surprisingly, then, we tend to take less responsibility when things go wrong. After all, we have bought the services of others to provide a solution. Any blame for ensuing problems can be placed on those whom we have hired. As we surrender autonomy, we take on frustration. Perhaps guilt, too, can drive us to find fault with caregivers who have not done their jobs well enough to satisfy us. Blame turns into lawsuits, which raise costs and lead to a defensive (proactive) approach to care, reflected in mounting regulations.

As for Betty Chang, she died peacefully in her sleep in her own home. Her daughter was at her side. A short time later, the family called me to "pronounce" her death and to sign the death certificate. Under the law, no one is allowed to die, even at home, unless a physician signs off on the event. I was more than happy to oblige. Over the years, I had come to trust and greatly respect Susie's dedication and care for her mother. Yet the choices she made do give rise to a few questions.

What if the Chang family had not found a physician willing to cooperate, one that insisted on aggressive care or on hospice care? There might have been legal ramifications. It is not unheard of for families to be reported to Adult Protective Services and investigated if they refuse institutional care for their elderly and rely instead on "unorthodox" methods of their own to take care of them.

As it was, Susie did accept and pay for help from medical professionals and from health care businesses whenever she needed respite from the care that she was offering her mother at home. Each time she did so, she received a new set of reasons as to why her mother should remain in the long-term care facility. No one seemed to understand Susie's refusal to relinquish responsibility for her mother.

The Question of Culture Change

The industry has taken some steps recently to make long-term care a bit more humane, if not luxurious. Almost seven years ago, one of the nursing homes in which I work adopted a "culture change" approach to improve life for its long-term residents. This facility has always been far and away the best of the fifty or so in which I have had patients, so I was excited at the prospect. Over time, however, it became clear that very little was really going to change. Except for the introduction of cats into the facility to amuse and comfort the residents, most alterations were cosmetic. The long-term care wings of the facility were renamed "family units." A few more parties and fundraising events took place than in the past, but that was about the extent of the new culture.

Meanwhile, the facility was hard at work marketing itself as a "pioneer" in long-term care, because it used a culture change model. The facility paid a rather large fee to a small public relations firm to teach its administrative staff how to capitalize on this feature when marketing the facility to prospective residents. Once the staff completed the PR company's training plan, the facility became a certified culture change provider.

All in all, I have been left with the impression that the culture change phenomenon is much like the trend in hospitals a decade or so ago to transform their maternity wards into "birthing centers," by wallpapering patient rooms and offering Mom and Dad champagne according to "hospital regulations."

Sadly, government regulations—well-intended though they may be—to protect vulnerable inhabitants from their corporate caregivers can inadvertently stymie true change. We are locked into managed care systems governed by law. It is no easy matter to institute change. The law must be brought along as well, and the law, as we know, moves slowly.

4

The Aging Experience

Aging can occur through what are termed normal processes. Or age can proceed in ways deemed pathological, though not at all uncommon.

Physical Changes

Normal Aging

- Weight loss
- Decreased strength
- Pain

Weight loss is a natural part of aging, unassociated with disease. Eating and chewing take longer, and the appetite decreases, as does food intake. Theory has it that the elder's metabolism slows to leave more food for the young. Regardless of the reason, the physiological change does occur: Typically, the elder needs very small portions to sustain life and maintain health.

Perversely enough, long-term care facilities gear their nutritional expectations to the needs of the young and active person. Indeed, most facilities seek to mold the elder into behaving as though he or she were a young adult, who eats heartily to maintain or even gain weight. Weight loss is taboo. Decreased appetite is treated as a medical emergency. Such expectations, however, are far from "normal" when it comes to aging, and this common misconception is unfortunate. I have seen many morbidly obese people finally lose some weight naturally in old age (which may enhance their ability to move about and function). Yet their very health improvements are then sabotaged, because they trigger a facility "care plan" to counteract the weight loss.

Decreased strength is also normal. Muscles have reduced resilience and stamina. The body has less reserve. Yet under normal circumstances, the elder should still be able to independently perform day-to-day functions, such as toileting, feeding, and walking, if at a slower rate than the younger person performs them.

Pain is a controversial issue. In my experience, it falls into two distinct categories, which should not be treated in the same way.

There is the anguish associated with natural processes such as birth, life's various stages (e.g., infancy, adolescence, midlife, aging) and death. Such pain brings with it increased insight and awareness, if it is successfully endured and overcome. No medical treatment is necessary.

Then there is pain associated with disease processes, such as arthritis and cancer. Such pain has no developmental benefit, and medicines and palliative interventions can be helpful.

Physical Changes
Pathological Aging

- Immobility
- Frequent falls
- Pain

Immobility. Although strength decreases with age—muscle mass diminishes and reaction times slow—total loss of mobility is not a normal result. Still, if and when immobility occurs, interventions, such as physical therapy, are available to help regain balance and strength. Medications can treat underlying causes, such as arthritis or the complications of diabetes and heart problems.

Frequent falls. In old age, balance is compromised, and eyesight and hearing are diminished, all of which can cause an occasional fall. The elder can adapt to such limitations. Sometimes medical and adjunct treatments are necessary to help reduce the number of falls, however. If frequent, falls can lead to fear of the associated pain and to an aversion to walking at all.

Pain. The type of pain associated with disease processes, such as arthritis and cancer, is pathological. Such pain provides no benefits and should be eased.

Emotional Changes
Normal Aging

- Short-term depression and grief

- Forgetfulness
- Introspection
- Fear

Short-term depression and grief. Some forms of depression and short-term grieving are normal. Short-term depression, such as that endured in adolescence or at mid-life, can be crucial to the development of our creativity and our capabilities. Such sadness forces us to reassess our lives. Similarly, grieving signals a time when we are working through the pain of our loss and learning from the experience. If anything, treating such forms of sadness as medical problems is detrimental to the developmental process and human creativity.

Minor depression is associated with losses and is characterized as a lack of dynamics in lifestyle. Moderate depression is associated with losses, decreased motivation, and perhaps some inability to continue with the daily routine. Pharmacological treatment of such early stages of depression is not a good idea. Depressed people need to have time to develop their own coping mechanisms before we intervene with medications. Medical relief may be short-lived, whereas the ways that individuals learn to cope on their own can serve them well through many hardships.

Is prolonged depression a natural part of aging? Probably not. More than likely, it is a maladaptive coping mechanism and contrary to survival. Severe depression is associated with loss of hope and perhaps vegetative symptoms, such as continuous sleeping and not eating. Prolonged grieving and depression should be carefully evaluated and treated appropriately.

Forgetfulness. Forgetfulness is common as we age. The mind has less reserve and forgetting helps us find room for more information and skills. Forgetting also is a way to cope with bad memories of painful events and losses in our lives. Because the elder has fewer responsibilities, and thus less to do and remember, memory loss does not necessarily pose a problem.

Introspection. The elder who keeps to himself, but is content and happy, is not in need of medical treatment. Losses can be so great that introversion is the only solution. Introspection can lead to productive outlets, such as travel, and to creative expression, such as writing. Yet it can also be expressed pathologically in such forms as psychosomatic disease or prolonged depression.

Fear. Fear, at least limited fear, is normal in many phases of the life cycle. It is natural to fear the unknown. Fear can encourage us to problem-solve, to try new things, and to take up new challenges.

Emotional Aging

Pathological Aging

- Prolonged depression and extended grief
- Paranoia
- Psychosis
- Severe memory loss or dementia

Prolonged depression and extended grief. When depression is prolonged and leads to alienation and profoundly negative personality changes, treatment should be considered. Pharmacological intervention to ease chronic depression is one of the most significant changes to have occurred in the practice of medicine over the past twenty years. Though such intervention can do wonders, its very impact means that it should be prescribed cautiously.

Long-term care facilities are a breeding ground for paranoia and psychosis. Clashing personality styles and sometimes vast differences in family background and social status can add to the impetus. Often a change in environment is the catalyst.

Paranoia. Paranoia is never normal. Rather it is a sign of mental and physical problems and always should be investigated and treated, if possible. Paranoia is unfortunately common among the elderly. Some elders with chronic mental illness have been paranoid for many years. In most cases, however, onset occurs in old age, and the elder has never before been paranoid. In such a state, an elder believes that somebody else is deliberately doing something for a reason that is meant to hurt him or her. Asked to give his children power of attorney, for example, he may believe that it is part of plan to kill him and steal his money. At the root of the condition is the affected individual's attempt to describe the actions of others (which are not understood) in his or her own terms. The condition is troublesome for all concerned—the individual, family, caregivers, and physician.

Psychosis. Like paranoia, psychosis is never normal. Yet it may be experienced for the first time in life once a person reaches old age. In a state of psychosis, a person sees, hears, or feels things that do not exist. As in the case of paranoia, the roots of psychosis lie in the attempt to cope with situations or circumstances that the person does not understand. An elder being bathed may experience staff assistance as sexual abuse. Elders may view door alarms and call lights as complex mechanisms created by the CIA to control their minds. Complicating matters, elders often are sensually impaired in terms of hearing, eyesight, and smell. They may well be mentally and physically impaired in other ways as well.

Severe Memory Loss or Dementia. Memory loss, when it is severe enough, can harm the individual and be considered pathological. A case in point is the inability to recognize family members. Although the available interventions remain limited, both medications and therapies can help reduce symptoms somewhat.

The Ages of Aging

Aging can be ascribed to three categories—the young-old, the middle-old, and the old-old. In a category all by themselves are the old-young—young people whose bodies have functionally aged as the result of disease or injury. In reality, of course, the aging process occurs along a continuum rather than in discrete episodes. Losses and gains are an integral part of the subphases to which individuals adapt as they pass through one or more of the categories.

The Old-Young (Eighteen to fifty-five)

These individuals have physical problems that make them functionally old. Their problems can result from chronic genetic disease processes, such as diabetes or multiple sclerosis, or from injury or other accident.

The Young-Old (Seventy-five to eighty-five)

Being young-old is precarious. The individual experiences physical changes that separate her from the younger person. Physical changes are most rapid during this phase. Health may begin to fail, and stamina decreases. Emotional losses occur as close friends, parents, or siblings become ill or die. At this stage, the elder often seeks to have one last chance at youth. Developing new activities that conform to physical limitations, or renewing old interests that were dormant for some time, are among the effective ways to cope. Denying the changes in oneself and blaming family members and professionals for losses, of course, are not.

The Middle-Old (Eighty-five to ninety-five)

This phase of aging is relatively quiet. Physical changes are less rapid. The middle-old tend to be more accepting. If well adjusted, they have grown accustomed to age. New activities and forms of satisfaction have been found to replace ones that are no longer possible.

The Old-Old (Ninety-five and above)

At this phase, the elder is resigned. Function again begins to decline dramatically. Change can occur very quickly. The body has few reserves, and all forms of stressors are traumatic. Once imminent, death cannot be delayed, though sometimes it can. Even at this late stage, exceptions occur.

A Long-Lived Life

Katie Collins lived to be 104. She first came to assisted living when she was about eighty. For the next five years, she had no problems other than ones that arise from what I call "wear and tear" aging. At eighty-five, Katie went to the hospital with acute abdominal pain. She did have a Living Will, but her wishes were somewhat vague.

She did not want permanent life support, but some interventions were acceptable. She had a small bowel obstruction that required surgery and a feeding tube inserted after surgery. Intended to be short term, the tube was to be removed once she recovered fully and was able to eat.

Although she did not recover enough to return to assisted living, Katie did regain her ability to eat on her own shortly after her admission to the nursing facility. After so much moving about, however, she had no desire to return to the hospital to have the feeding tube removed. As a rule, the tube went unused. The exceptions were her medicines, which she did not like to taste, so the nurses put them in her tube. During the course of what turned out to be close to another decade, neither Mrs. Collins nor her family updated her Living Will, although the staff and I brought the matter up from time to time.

When Mrs. Collins was ninety-five, she had a massive stroke. She was hospitalized and stabilized but regained no independent functions. In a vegetative state, she survived through tube feeding. Once she returned to the facility, her feeding tube was to remain in permanent use.

Katie was a private-pay resident. Neither insurance, Medicare, nor Medicaid paid for her stay in the facility. Instead it was her family who paid upward of eight thousand dollars a month for her stay.

When Mrs. Collins reached 102, six years after her stroke, her daughter, Alice, asked to speak with me. Alice (who was eighty at the time) did not think that the right decisions had been made with respect to her mother. Now she wanted to know if I could stop all her medications except for comfort from pain.

"I don't wish for mother to live on just because she's on medications—not that I want to stop the tube feedings or put her in hospice care, mind you."

I tended to agree, and brought her request up with the facility staff. Everyone was comfortable with Alice Collins' desires for her mother's care.

I stopped Mrs. Collins' medications. She experienced no adverse consequences and continued to receive her tube feedings. She developed no new medical problems and continued to do well. Two years passed. Katie turned 104. Again, her daughter wanted to speak with me.

"My husband has lung disease," she said as she sat down with me to talk. "We're moving to Florida to help him avoid the winters and live longer." She gave me a long look.

"I'm sorry to hear about his disease," I said. "You must be concerned about what to do about your mother."

"That's right," she nodded. Then she gave me another long look and sighed. "Do you suppose the tube feeding should be stopped? I'd like to be with Mother at the end," Alice went on quietly. "I sure don't want to leave her alone, but I don't have much choice, what with Henry's condition."

"I certainly understand," I said to her.

"There's another thing, Doctor. My mother's funds are nearly exhausted. We'll have to apply for state assistance pretty soon."

By then, Katie Collins had spent twenty-five years in a long-term care facility.

"Tube feedings or not, I don't imagine that she has much time left," Alice said

Her mother was 104, after all. The life cycle was near completion, regardless of feedings or medicine. At this point, sustenance had become a legal issue. I consulted with the facility's Ethics Committee, as well as with hospice caregivers.

The tube feedings were stopped.

Shortly thereafter, Mrs. Collins died peacefully. Alice was at her side.

A Woman of Spirit

How people experience aging is a combination of the actual process and their perception of it. A person's attitude or spirit is a combination of personality and experience. Older people retain the same personality that they had in youth. Only advanced dementia or extreme physical illness will alter it. Hope Brown is a prime example of someone who never lost her spirit. Eighty when I met her, she suffered from end-stage pulmonary disease, cardiac disease, and arthritis. To survive, she depended on oxygen as well as on many other medications. In and out of the hospital as well as the nursing home to convalesce after surgeries, eventually she would make her way home again to her apartment in an independent-living complex that served meals.

Each time she went to the hospital, she became a bit weaker. Each time she returned home, there was one less thing that she could do for herself. Attitude in her case made all the difference. Although she valued her independence, she also realized that she needed the support of others. She hired home care staff to come and help her. She had a very supportive daughter, Anna, who managed her finances and medications and who came to visit several times a week.

For some time, Mrs. Brown continued her pattern of going into the hospital, convalescing at Fern Oakes, the LTC facility where I first met her, and finally returning home to her independent-living complex. Because Hope had trouble traveling to her physician's office, I agreed to be her doctor and to pay house calls to her apartment, something I rarely do on account of time constraints and legal issues. I made the exception in this case, because I trusted the family (in this case, Anna) to call me when needed, yet not abuse my services. As it was, I never charged for seeing Hope when she was at home. The insurance situation was just too complicated to make it worth the trouble.

Eventually, she became so debilitated that her days consisted of mustering up the energy to take care of her basic needs. Still continent, she could no longer walk to the bathroom. By relying on adult diapers, she remained able to attend to personal hygiene herself. Facility policy required residents to eat at least two meals in the dining room every day to remain in the independent living complex. For a little while longer, she managed to get to the dining room for lunch, but the time came when she could no longer make it for dinner. Although Hope had no cognitive deficits, her breathing was so compromised that she could no longer live within the rules.

With mixed feelings, she moved into Fern Oakes. Alongside her resignation was the pride in making her own decision to come live here, as well as relief. She had struggled on her own for some time. As for Fern Oakes, she had rehabilitated there often enough to almost think of it as her second home. She liked many of the staff members, and she enjoyed the food served there, especially breakfast. Hope went on to live several more pleasant and productive years. She fit into the facility, adjusted well, and developed a daily routine.

A Day in the Life

An early riser—Hope awoke at five—she headed down to the hall bathroom, where she toileted and sponge-bathed herself. This exertion took her about an hour and sometimes fatigued her so much that she went back to bed. There she read a little and listened to music.

After breakfast in her room, she spent an hour watching a religious program on television. She prayed and took a nap for a few hours. At about ten a.m., she awoke again. A nurse's aide helped her dress. By eleven, she would call her daughter. At eleven-thirty, she would begin the long march in her wheeled walker to the main dining room for lunch. (Everywhere that Hope went, her can of oxygen was sure to go, she used to joke.) The travel distance of about one thousand feet took her twenty or thirty minutes to complete. About half-way there, she would stop at the nursing station to rest and chat, and perhaps take a sip from her water bottle. On the final leg of her journey, she would stop again to speak with residents and staff whom she passed in the halls. Yet she nearly always managed to arrive in the dining room before lunch was served. After she ate, she rested at the table for a little while in preparation for the return trek.

Back in her room, she would nap for about an hour and then get up to join in one of the afternoon activities, such as bingo or crafts. Three times a week she would go to an exercise activity in the therapy room with a few other residents. She worked to keep what little physical function she had left. Through physical therapy, combined with assistance from the nursing staff, she actually became more independent than when she lived in her apartment by herself. Eventually, she was able to get to the dining room twice daily, something she had lost the capacity to do in assisted living.

At about five, Mrs. Brown would return to her room and prepare for dinner. She would go to the bathroom, wash up, and sit down to rest before her second walk to the dining room. At this point in her day, she had little appetite but ate her meal anyway. Fatigued, she was often brought back to her room in a wheelchair. She would lie in bed and read a bit. Her daughter would call her again and chat.

Evening activities varied. Sometimes Hope would listen to music. Other times she would watch television. Occasionally she would go out again and spend time in activities with other residents. Several times a week, a movie was shown in the main activity room, where snacks and drinks were served. Several times a month, outside entertainment, such as a local choir or a chamber ensemble, would come to perform. Whenever Hope felt up to them, she enjoyed these performances.

By ten o'clock, she was tired. She was washed, changed, and put to bed. Several times during the night, a nurse would wake her so that she could take her medications and undergo some prescribed breathing treatments.

Again, it would be five a.m. Hope would start her routine. She maintained this daily regimen for nearly three years.

Only for financial reasons did I recommend that she be enrolled in hospice care. Her daughter, Anna, was starting to have trouble paying for her mother's oxygen. Hospice would pay for the tanks and could also offer a more comfortable bed than the family could afford. The decision to enter hospice care was hard on Hope.

"You're no worse off than you were yesterday," I assured her. "We just want to give you more care, so that you'll be more comfortable."

Still, I could not soften the blow entirely. "The move into hospice care doesn't mean that you will die soon," I explained. "But it does mean that you are entering the final phase of your life."

"I don't want to admit that I'm dying," she told me.

Hope lived under hospice care for another two years. She had bouts of pneumonia and suffered several falls and minor injuries, but she kept her mental faculties intact and was able to move about slowly and thereby exert some independence. I visited her monthly and almost always found her in a good mood. Clearly she had found the resources to accept where she was in her life.

My goal during these visits was to support her own positive outlook with the encouragement that some aspects of her care and life could be made better. I did not offer Hope a cure. I did stress simple changes that would allow her to reach for attainable goals.

A Life Well Lived

Recounting a day in the life of a nursing home patient such as Hope Brown says little about her as an individual, except perhaps to speak to her determination and grit. I was fortunate enough, however, to come to know Hope as one of the most admirable of all my patients. I came to see her as exemplary, not only in aging successfully but in living the kind of life that makes successful aging that much more likely.

Hope Brown was an only child. She lived in a small and rural community, where houses stood on acres of land, far apart from one another. As a little girl, she would spend her days drawing princesses in colorful outfits. She dreamt of being a princess herself. A bit lonely, she built on her dreams, just as she built on her ability to draw and design clothes.

As a young woman, she learned to sew and to make her own wardrobe, as well as to sew items made to order for her friends and family. After high school she earned enough money to go to art school, but World War II intervened. She had to drop out to support her family. After the war, when Hope and her husband had more money, she used her disposable income to augment her creativity. As her children grew, so did her ideas. She made prom dresses, unique party food, and creative decorations for bat mitzvahs and other festive occasions.

Once her children were grown, she had more free time. Friends and family encouraged her to market her skills. At first she took some pieces of her handmade clothing to consignment shops, where they sold quickly. Then she spotted a demand for upscale clothing for infants and toddlers and for designs with a practical twist. She began to sketch items that were easy to launder yet attractive. Her clothing was designed to make breastfeeding and diapering easy to do. In time Hope opened her own store, then a mail order catalog, and, finally, an Internet website. Delighted and proud of her business, Hope did not bask long. At this point, her husband was in poor health and needed care. Her own eyesight was failing, as was her health in general from years of tobacco use.

Still, she proved just how well she could adjust. She sold her business to a large department store chain but kept consulting fees for her future ideas. Proceeds from the sale paid for some home care for her husband and some respite for her. Now she could spend some of her days writing up her creations (In time, these notes became a book). The arrangement left her quite content. She and Jim were even able to go on a couple of cruises before he passed away.

Not only her husband but many of her friends died over the next few years. She took solace in making a quilt—unique to each of them—incorporating a scrap or two of fabric from their home furnishings or clothing to help express who each of these people were and what they had meant to her.

Even after she moved into the assisted-living apartment complex, she continued consulting through the Internet. No longer able to see well enough to quilt, she found a computer program to help her with the stitching. She also organized a group of ladies in the building to help sew the pieces together. When she was in the hospital with recurrent problems that stemmed from her lung disease, her daughter stepped in to manage her consulting business for her.

At Fern Oakes she could not see to sew, but she could still think. Her roommate, who was incontinent and demented, would put her hands in her diaper and dirty herself. Mrs. Brown had an idea. In fact, she had several. She designed a number of outfits (similar to ones in her children's clothing line). One of her creations was an overall with a zipper in the legs and crotch, which not only took care of the hygiene issue but made for a nice-looking suit, which the roommate as well as other residents could wear without worries. Family members and caregivers liked these designs enough to help sew the outfits. When it was discovered that another resident was allergic to disposable diapers, Hope designed easy-wash, cloth diapers to fit a number of sizes.

Once she entered hospice care, her mind began to slow.

"My ideas have come to an end," she told me.

When several women expressed an interest in her lifetime of

skills, however, she agreed to lead an activity group to impart some advice and instruction on sewing and clothing design.

Hope had good days and bad days, but she always rebounded. I never thought she would die. Her health problems were chronic conditions and had become so stable, that I almost forgot about them. Whenever I saw her, I enjoyed her spirit and stamina and the stories she told me about her life, which had been hard at times but also tremendously rewarding. She lived her life according to her dreams, skills, and abilities. Even now in hospice, she was sharing what she knew. She was creating a legacy of skills and knowledge for others to keep and use.

One day, Hope went into a rapid decline. She had dinner and went to bed early. She did not wake as usual. The staff tried to rouse her, but she only groaned a bit. For several days she ate nothing and took only a few sips of water. Most probably she had had a stroke.

On the morning of the third day, I went in to see her. I knew that she was dying and signaled as much to the staff. That evening she did die, surrounded by her daughter, several staff members, and the hospice nurse at her bedside. I was not there, however. I could not bring myself to say goodbye. I had grown to admire her too much. There was no way that I could have hidden the great pain I felt at her passing. Hope was my role model for the life well lived. She knew how to adjust, not only to changes in circumstances but also to changes in herself—physical, social, emotional, and mental. She never forgot her interests or lost her personal style. For a few crazy hours, I refused to accept that she was really dead.

My memories of Hope remain scarred by that day when I was unable to say goodbye. A month passed before I could send a note to Anna. *Your mother had such an impact on my life*, I wrote. *She did not lose her spirit.*

A Quiet End

A loss of spirit need not mean a fall from grace, however. It may simply signal the quiet end to a normal life, lived fully and satisfactorily. In that regard, I think of Darla Smithers, who passed through the "young-old" years of her life with few medical problems. She lived independently until the age of eighty-seven when her daughters moved her into Fern Oakes after hospitalization for a urinary tract infection.

Despite her robust health and freedom from disease, it was clear why her daughters had moved their mother into the nursing home.

Darla showed signs of wear-and-tear aging when she came into my care. Despite the lack of medical problems, such as coronary disease and diabetes, she found it difficult to see, to hear, and to walk. Yet her mind was largely intact but for some forgetfulness. She still had her strong spirit and a good-hearted, if tough-minded, personality.

"Mom worked hard all her life," Debby, the eldest daughter, told me. "She had a long career as a surgical nurse, starting way back in the 1940s. For a married woman, that kind of thing was unheard of in her day."

"She came from a long line of country doctors," Ellie, the younger girl joined in to say. "Her dad was a physician in rural Kentucky. So was our own dad."

"Daddy died ten years ago," Debby wanted me to know.

In the months that followed, I grew to admire Darla's daughters. Both women were attentive and supportive of their mother's needs. They were involved in her care and were her advocates. They called me when necessary, were not abusive of my time, and respected my opinion. I also respected theirs.

Wear-and-tear aging caused Darla a cascade of new problems, as did the transition from independent living to nursing home care. She could not walk, yet wanted to be independent. She fell several times attempting to get to the toilet. Luckily, she did not experience any prolonged injury, such as a hip fracture. Because of her limited ability to see and to hear, a caregiver began to come in and help her bathe and dress. This sort of personal assistance went against Darla's grain. At first wary, she grew paranoid about the motives of the people who surrounded her. She began to have nightmares and no longer participated in communal activities as she had when she first arrived at Fern Oakes several months previously.

Mrs. Smithers' daughters were quick to express concern. When they came in to speak with me, they handed me a written list:

- Mom was on too many medications, which might be leading to her confusion.
- Mom needed therapy so that she could walk again.
- Mom needed cataract surgery so that she would be able to see again.

- Mom needed to get out and do activities so that she would become more interested in life.

"All of these concerns are perfectly valid," I told the two women. "Let's address them and see if we can help your mother."

I began by gradually reducing Mrs. Smithers' medications. She experienced no adverse effects but did not seem less disoriented, either. Physical therapy led to greater mobility, although Darla still could not walk. Cataract surgery improved her sight to some extent. Most gratifying was the lift in her spirits that occurred, perhaps as a result of the various interventions. Mrs. Smithers did adjust to the facility and eventually began to join in some of the activities. She liked to bowl from her wheelchair, and her sure hand with a paint brush impressed us all. No longer paranoid, she enjoyed constant praise for her watercolors.

Debby and Ellie continued to wonder why their mom could not walk.

"Is Mom in pain?" Ellie asked.

"Pain could hinder her therapy," I agreed.

I placed Darla on a mild arthritic drug. This drug had few side effects but could cause stomach bleeding, especially in the elderly.

Mrs. Smithers became weaker. At first, her daughters and I thought that she might be depressed. I had discontinued her antidepressant a few months back. The counselor who came in to examine her said otherwise, however. As Mrs. Smithers grew weaker, I ordered blood and diagnostic tests. The tests showed that she had become dangerously anemic. Perhaps anemia was a side effect of her arthritic medication? Mrs. Smithers was admitted to the hospital, where her treatment was prolonged by complications.

Not surprisingly, she developed bedsores (decubiti) in the hospital, and when she finally did return to the facility, she was bed-bound and very deconditioned. The advance practice nurse, who specialized in skin wounds, saw her and recommended a feeding tube for nutrition.

"Her wounds won't heal otherwise," the nurse said. "She's not eating enough to sustain herself and to heal at the same time."

Her daughters agreed to the feeding tube.

After the procedure, Mrs. Smithers did show a certain

improvement physically. She was in no pain, her wounds healed a bit, and she was eating "pleasure foods" by mouth. Debby and Ellie hired private sitters to watch over their mother nearly twenty-four hours a day.

Although Darla was alive, clearly she had lost her spirit. Her eyes looked out at the world vacantly. Her wonderful smile appeared only rarely now.

Her two daughters took in the change quietly. This time they brought me no list of concerns. Their mother was aged, and she was dying. They had done their best to give her quality of life at the end of her life.

5

LTC — The Ever-Shifting Scene

Monday continues, as do my rounds.

It is about 8:30 a.m. as I drive to my next facility, Sweet Penny Tree, twenty minutes away from Apple Lane. I come to this facility several times a week. Until recently, it has been one of my favorite places to go. Not anymore. Things are changing. A new administrator and a director of nursing have been hired. Their key agenda seems to be to fire every staff member who has worked here for more than three years, regardless of skill level. I have no idea why, although an unsatisfactory profit margin is probably the reason at bottom. The long-term care industry is highly competitive, and it is quite common for a facility to try to attract more business by changing its name and management, sometimes almost overnight.

This industry phenomenon can make the idea of "place" somewhat elusive at times. I remember one weekend when I was asked to respond to an emergency. The voice message on my pager went something like this:

"We've got an emergency here at—. Wait a minute, please."

I could hear my caller's voice turn away from the telephone to speak to a colleague.

"Sylvia, what's the name of this place?"

"Colmes Manor," came the reply.

My caller redirected her voice into the phone. "Sorry about that. I'm just here this weekend, from an agency. Colmes Manor. That's where I am."

The temp hung up, unaware that the facility was no longer doing business under that name. Luckily, I had an old phone directory. If the name of the facility had changed, the phone number had not.

No image makeover is needed at Sweet Penny Tree. If I have loved this facility, it is largely because of the devoted and capable staff. Perhaps the new owners simply wish to mark their new turf. In any case, the termination of good people leaves me depressed and confused. The residents are suffering.

I drive into the lot and barely find a parking space. New construction is under way. Corporate consultants (who work for the company that owns the facility) are visiting to review records. The first person I see on the way into the building is Eva, a resident I care for. She is slumped on a park bench, asleep, despite the gentle rain that has begun to fall. A few other residents linger out in the cold, huddled under the awning, puffing on cigarettes. They all greet me, including those who are not my patients. A few of them ask to see me today. I tell them to go to their rooms and wait.

Inside I urge the receptionist to bring Eva in out of the rain, which she is quick to do. As I move through the halls, I am greeted cordially by everyone except the new administrator and the director of nursing who seem to duck back into their offices to avoid me. I meet with the nursing supervisors and some of the floor nurses, who have a list of requests ready for me. They have not called me all weekend, except to verify orders on one new admission, knowing that I will be here today.

I see the new resident and several others, who need or want to be seen for a variety of reasons, many of them not medical. One resident asks for a private consultation to describe the bad food. I listen but explain that the kitchen and dining room are not my domains. Another woman needs ten minutes to reminiscence about Ernie, her late husband, just as she does every week, though she is not technically my patient. These are the types of visits that I always do "pro bono," out of respect for the need that we all have for common-sense advice and reassurance.

I look for the few charts to update. They are missing, in use by the corporate record consultants. The medical records director retrieves them for me. I fill in the charts and prepare to leave.

In the hallway, I run into two long-time members of the staff— Marlin—a tall, dark nurse—and Joan—a short, round dietician. Both are highly competent. They are assets to the facility.

"Someone is spreading rumors about us," Joan tells me. "I think we'll be pushed out."

Marlin smiles but looks uncomfortable. He is not one for frank talk, though he fears for his job as much as she does.

"Oh, well," Joan sighs. "Maybe Tammy will come back and throw us a party." She gives me a wink.

All three of us smile now.

Joan is referring to Tammy Shest, a former resident, known for hosting many a party to say good-bye to staff.

Putting Up a Fight

I remember the first time that I met Tammy Shest. She sat in her wheelchair as if on a throne and blocked the corridor as if that were to be expected.

"Take a good look at these legs," she commanded, pointing to the inert limbs, large and swollen from previous heart failure, encased in woolen kneesocks above broad feet, propped solidly on the foot rests of the stainless steel chair.

With barely a glance at her legs, my eyes panned up to meet hers: clear ice-blue, intelligent and fierce.

"I used to wear shorts in the summer," she growled, "just like you do." Somehow it was my fault that she no longer did. What was I going to do to about it? Her tone of voice accused me.

"You got to fix me up, Doctor! That's your job."

Ms. Shest was seventy-five when she arrived at Sweet Penny Tree, plagued by severe lung disease, as well as coronary disease. An electric wheelchair allowed her to roam the halls of the facility and get outside to smoke her pack of Marlboros.

Only "yesterday," Tammy was beautiful, personable, and had her whole life ahead of her. She had dreams. She could do anything, and her promise would last. In the meantime, she drank, she smoked, and she ate what she wanted. She worked some but saved no money. She had many boyfriends but was waiting for Mr. Right to start a family. Mr. Right never materialized.

Now she cast her cold eye on the "old folks" who surrounded her. "I am not that old," she scoffed. "I am not that pathetic. As God is my judge, I am going to wake up from this nightmare," she would say, as she pounded the armrests of her chair. What was happening to her body could not be true.

Only of course it was true. Her health was poor. She could not breathe without oxygen and was unable to walk, except from the bed to the wheelchair and from the wheelchair to the toilet. She depended on medications to regulate her blood sugar, blood pressure, and breathing. Physical limitations and dependence on others were a special hardship for a free spirit. She could no longer do as she pleased.

Much later, when we knew each other better, Ms. Shest confessed to me quietly in the privacy of her room: "I never thought I would get old so fast! There must be a way back," she would murmur—that was her mantra—a way back to being her former self, beautiful and vibrant again. If only she could find the right pill. In pursuit of rejuvenation, she went to specialists and had numerous tests done in hospitals. Why could she not walk or breathe? Sure, cigarettes and junk food were not good for you—but could they really do this much damage?

She blamed the hospital. She blamed the physical therapists. She blamed the physicians who cared for her. Okay, so she continued to smoke. At times, she skipped her medications. The bottom line was, the rest of us had failed her. We had not done our jobs. We had not made her better.

She was especially belligerent toward me.

"Why haven't you cured me, Doctor?"

"I can offer you several possible treatments," I explained, "but I have no cures."

She stared at me, dead-eyed. "I should fire you," she said. "I should get another doctor."

"That's your choice," I said. She still had some power.

For quite a long time, Ms. Shest remained intent on finding a way out of Sweet Penny Tree. She was good on the phone and knew how to persist in making inquiries to find a suitable apartment, but her options were too limited, given her financial status.

When she ran out of tests to take and real estate listings to pursue, she became depressed and withdrawn. She had come to an impasse. She had hit a wall. There she stayed. My weekly talks with her led to little more than another threat to fire me.

Imperceptibly, however, she was undergoing a deep-seated change. After many months, I began to see signs of adjustment. During this time, we got word that several of her friends outside the facility had passed away. At last she seemed to come to a decision, to make peace with her life as it was, in the here and now. She began to accept the help that I could offer. More remarkably still, she began to accept some responsibility for her failing health, to own up to the fact that smoking for many years had contributed to, if not caused, her disease. She could admit that her problems were not simply the result of the total incompetence of the entire medical profession.

She made some effort to help herself. She smoked a little less, and her breathing improved. She gained enough stamina to walk a bit.

The time came when she actually apologized.

"I'm sorry I've been so nasty," she told me.

I remembered the day when we first met and the spark of fury in her eyes.

Life of the Party

Once Ms. Shest made up her mind that she was there to stay, she threw herself into life at Sweet Penny Tree. She had a private room on the first floor, which made it easy for her to wheel herself outside to smoke and to catch the bus to run errands. Eventually she would go out to dinner with her new friends, including a gentleman with whom she enjoyed flirting.

As a natural born leader, Tammy put her sense of command to use. She organized the residents to form a council, so that they might have a say in how administrators managed the facility. If she never did find a way back to being eighteen, she had learned to meet life halfway and then some. As a result, she was able to make many improvements in the life that she and her friends led at Sweet Penny Tree. She would tell me when people were ill and needed to be seen. She organized parties of all kinds, including her famous farewell get-togethers for departing staff.

Then, after nearly two years at the facility, the last of which had been such a triumph, life was no longer ready to meet her in quite the same way.

The new administrator, who now worried Marlin and Joan, upset Tammy first. One of the first things he did after he arrived was to reassign some of the resident rooms. Tammy was moved to the second floor. She was not pleased. Being wheelchair-bound on the second floor cramped her style, she told him. She was not able to get outside as easily anymore, and she missed her former neighbors, now her friends.

The administrator listened politely but did nothing.

As his assistant explained to me later, the reassignments were to attract new residents to the "nicer" rooms. This strategy made good business sense. The resident's room, after all, is the last bastion of the personal life. Here the resident sets out a few family photos, and perhaps a few pieces of furniture and favorite objects, vestiges of a life of seventy years or more.

In a huff, Ms. Shest reverted to form. For once I could sympathize. She made calls to several other long-term care facilities. She found one that she thought she would like and arranged her transfer there. A leader to the end, she convinced three other residents to leave Sweet Penny Tree with her.

Mourned in Style

As I was to learn later, Tammy did not adjust well to her new home. The residents there never really accepted her, put off by her take-charge manner in what was a well-settled social landscape.

"I'm an outsider," she told me, when I visited her.

"That will change," I said, to encourage her. "Join in the activities."

She nodded, but she looked glum. The old fire seemed banked. The move from one facility to another had exhausted her.

In fact, Ms. Shest became quite depressed. She had neither the energy nor sufficient support from the facility staff to get help to deal with her mixture of sadness and anger. No longer her doctor, I kept track of her through a colleague of mine, which is how I learned that she was in and out of the hospital with pneumonia. She did return to the new nursing home facility for several months but never did form any ties there. She developed a skin wound from bedsores that required surgery.

Ms. Shest passed away suddenly about a month later. My colleague let me know. Her funeral was a solitary event. Not so the memorial service at Sweet Penny Tree. We her friends, who had lived and worked with her, mourned her death in a style that Tammy would have approved. We threw a real party—those of us, that is, still there to remember her. By that time, Joan and Marlin were long gone.

Not a Medical Problem

This morning I leave Sweet Penny Tree by a side door to avoid the main entrance. (There is always one more resident posted there to ask me a question.) In the parking lot, I see that an earth mover has blocked my car. I must return to the main entrance, after all, and ask the receptionist to page someone for assistance. Ten minutes later, a worker strolls along the driveway. Reluctantly, he moves the vehicle to let me out.

As I drive off, I receive a call on my cell phone. It is Thelma Lewis, a nurse at Sweet Penny Tree.

"Something happened here this weekend that I should've told you about when you were here, but I couldn't figure out how to say it exactly." She sounds embarrassed. "Two residents were caught attempting sex." She tells me their names. Both of them are under my care. "There was no real problem, but we've written it up as a resident-to-resident altercation."

I laugh. "Well, you're right. Sex is not usually a medical problem." On impulse, I could not help but add: "I hope their attempt is more successful next time."

Over the phone, Thelma's intake of breath is audible. Clearly she was not expecting my remark, but what she says next shows that she is willing to reconsider her attitude.

"Maybe we take everything too seriously around here," she allows. Then I hear her giggle. "What with Steve Harper involved, I would've bet on success the first time around."

"I see what you mean," I say to Thelma. Steve Harper is no little old man. At about fifty years of age, he is the resident sex symbol.

I say good-bye to Thelma and switch off my cell to negotiate city traffic. As I drive, I try and recall what I know of Steve Harper from our few conversations since he arrived at Sweet Penny Tree about six months ago.

Steve had a history of drug and alcohol use, which led to a couple of falls more than a decade ago. The first time that he fell and hit his head, he had internal bleeding that required neurosurgery. He experienced residual memory loss but could take care of his own needs. A few months later, he fell and hit his head again. This time the damage was more dramatic. He required repeat surgery and was on life support for some time. He did go home eventually, but his injuries seriously compromised his memory and impulse control. Not long after that, he got into a fight in a bar, where someone else got badly hurt. He came to us straight out of prison, where he had done about ten years of time.

Before his accident, Steve told me that he had made his living as a fashion photographer for high-profile magazines, such as *Glamour* and *Cosmopolitan*. When times were tough, he supplemented his income as a bartender. Even after the accident and imprisonment, he could have passed for a "GQ" model himself. Tall and muscular, he had dark, soulful eyes and thick, curly hair. Half the staff had a crush on him, as did many of the elderly women residents. Age had not diminished their ability to appreciate sex appeal, even if all they could manage to do was look.

Sex Is Good

Much later, Joan (the dietician who feared for her job at Sweet Penny Tree) would fill me in on the sexual escapade, which Thelma had reported so haltingly. According to Joan, Steve Harper claimed not to have had sex during the ten years he spent in prison. Be that as it may, he was choosy about his encounters with women and not about to take up with just anyone.

Recently, a new resident had come to live at Sweet Penny Tree, who apparently met Steve's standards. In her late forties, Antoinette had a nice figure (including breast implants) and was "very coquettish and experienced," Joan told me. She had a history of chronic mental illness and diabetes.

"Still, she's definitely good looking, Joan said. "Besides that, she's a fine artist. She spends her days painting in oils. She's done a great portrait of Steve.

"Well, to get to the point," Joan went on to say, Steve and Tony finally had their "honeymoon." Behind closed doors, they attempted to get to know each other a bit better. As they did, quite a lot of noise could be heard emanating from Steve's room. The certified nursing assistants on the floor at the time feared that either Steve or his roommate had fallen or in some other way had injured himself. Without bothering to knock, the two young women burst through the door. Of course they upset the couple, in flagrante delicto. According to the two nursing assistants, however, Steve tumbled off the bed before anything had actually "happened."

Steve and Tony have since gone on to establish themselves as a happy couple at Sweet Penny Tree, where they continue to reside in a locked behavioral unit. Nowadays they no longer attempt sex—they have succeeded many times. Their main issue these days is jealousy among the other men: Tony has strayed a few times, but Steve always forgives her. Luckily for them, the current administrator tolerates discreet sexual activity between consenting adults—Thelma's good-natured prudery notwithstanding.

Prison Is Better

Steve has continued to be a patient of mine, and I have visited him weekly over many years. Despite his lucidness, his brain injury does not allow him to realize that he has repeated the same things to me over and over.

Every time that I see him, he compares the LTC facility with prison.

"The food is better here, and I can have a girlfriend, but otherwise it's the same. I hardly ever get the hell out of here. The outings are only once every three months, and they take us to dumb places. Even if they went somewhere interesting, I have almost no money—maybe ten dollars a week—and I get no chance to earn any." (It is true that the rest of his disability payment must go to the nursing home for his room and board.) "If nothing else, I could wait tables. I already paid my dues and did my time—so why I am here?"

Typical of his type of brain damage, he begins to ramble. "I tell you, it's just like jail. Only worse. At least there they had a gym. I could smoke anywhere I wanted to. I could hang out at the library. Besides, prison was free."

"That's not so," I tell him every time.

Still, I am always struck by Steve's comparison, which does make me stop and think.

Do we offer residents what they need? Sometimes yes and sometimes no. In a nutshell, here is what they need, and here is what at a minimum they can expect to get—the most that long-term care institutions can guarantee.

They need food.

They get nutrition.

They need personal attention and help with the basic activities of daily living.

They receive physical assistance from hired staff.

They need human interaction and stimulation.

They are protected by legal regulations against negligent care.

They need treatment for illness and alleviation of physical and mental pain.

They get administrative plans for their care.

They need the finances to cover basic needs.

They have insurance or they qualify for state support.

Sometimes a good match occurs between what the resident needs and what the facility offers. Too often, however, needs are met by poor substitutes for what would truly be fulfilling. Just because a facility's kitchen provides good nutrition, for example, does not mean that it offers satisfying or delicious meals.

Like a prison, the long-term care facility is a public domain, which constrains its inhabitants in many different ways. Unlike a prison, the LTC has no punitive intent, though some residents may feel punished anyway. How the facility manages the aging experience obviously can influence the individual's success in doing the same.

6

Mrs. Jamison and the Care Team

It takes many people to make up what is known as a care team. As a whole, this team can determine the culture and the quality of life to be had at a long-term care facility. In my experience, a care team's temperament can even help determine who resides in the facility during a given period of time, by attracting a certain kind of person and his or her family. In general, the care team can be characterized in the following ways:

- The normal care team
- The bickering (dysfunctional) care team
- The threatening care team
- The absent care team
- The passive care team
- No care team

The Professional Family

Typically, **administrative staff** oversee the day-to-day business of the long-term care facility, as well as the yearly on-site surveys by inspectors to ensure that the many regulations that govern nursing homes are met. Repeat surveys are not uncommon in the same year to address complaints. A survey that results in a substandard rating can lead to both fines and modifications by the sanctioned facility.

When it comes to actual caregiving, **nursing assistants** help residents perform basic bodily functions and hygiene. A **floor nurse** gives residents their medications, assesses their physical state, and provide treatments, such as wound care. Typically, such a nurse is responsible for some twenty-five residents per shift. A **nursing supervisor** is usually in direct contact with physicians regarding medical care, in addition to overseeing nursing. An **ancillary nurse** provides the proper documentation on each resident. In what is largely an administrative role, the **director of nursing** oversees the nursing staff and is involved in evaluating quality assurance.

He or she assesses ancillary services, such as laboratory work and pharmaceutical provision, and may be involved in assessing residents prior to admission to determine their appropriateness for the facility.

In addition to the **physicians** who provide medical care to residents, specialists such as podiatrists, optometrists, psychiatrists, and physiatrists may visit the facility to provide specialized medical care. A doctor also serves as the facility's **medical director**. He or she oversees facility medical issues, which may include legal matters, and ensures facility compliance with proper medical care. Often the director is the personal physician of at least a third of the residents.

The care team may also include **physical/occupational** and **speech therapists**. These professionals help residents regain function after a stroke, fracture, or other injury, and also help them to retain certain functions, such as walking and performing personal hygiene.

A **social worker** provides a sounding board for resident complaints and guidance on family and financial issues; he or she plans discharge. A **psychologist** speaks with residents who are feeling depressed or having adjustment problems; he or she may see residents on a regular basis but does not prescribe medications.

To function at all, a long-term care facility depends on **support staff**, in addition to administrative and medical staff. A **beautician** can greatly enhance a resident's sense of well-being with a hair style and manicure as much or more than a counselor can with a therapy session or a psychiatrist with an antidepressant. **Launderers**, too, can make a difference in the quality of life; in their case by properly caring for residents' clothing so that it is not ruined or lost. **Maintenance crews** are needed to do repairs, and **housekeepers** to clean. These staff members have daily contact with the residents, which can lead to pleasant socializing and sometimes friendships. Likewise, the quality of the food, which **nutritionists** and **dietary specialists** choose, and **cooks** and **kitchen aides** prepare, for residential snacks and meals makes a significant difference one way or the other. Enjoying a meal can be one of the few sensual pleasures remaining to an individual. **Activities personnel** plan and supervise daily diversions (crafts and games) and outings (to museums, concerts, shopping malls) as well as parties and other social gatherings within the facility. **Volunteers** and **clergy** offer companionship and comfort to some.

All of these people come together to form the care team. As mentioned above, the interpersonal dynamics that develop among them often lead to a collective characterization of the team as normal, bickering, threatening, absent, passive, or nonexistent altogether. To understand the impact of each type of team, consider a former patient of mine, Rose Jamison, who encountered all six types of care teams over the course of four years at an upscale facility.

Mrs. Jamison came to Sonoma Ranch when she was eighty-two years old and had advanced Parkinson's disease. She had lived with Julie, the eldest of her two daughters, for about five years before they reached a mutual decision that she should come to Sonoma for long-term care.

When she arrived at the facility, a smartly dressed daughter stood on either side of her wheelchair. As Julie and her sister, Emma, arranged their mother's new room, Mrs. Jamison directed them to set a photo of themselves on top of her chest of drawers. The picture was taken when the two were in preschool and dressed in identical pink pinafores, which their mother had sewn herself.

Rose (as she liked us to call her) appeared likely to adjust well to her new surroundings. Despite the Parkinson's, her health was stable and otherwise good. Her mind was lucid and alert, and among her belongings were a number of mystery novels and a game of Scrabble.

Yet, before very long, an odd pattern in her behavior emerged. Every few weeks, Rose took to her bed for no apparent reason. From there, she would sound the alarm and telephone her daughters, then head off to the emergency room. On calmer days, she would merely complain to me. Though I could find nothing wrong, I made appointments for her to see multiple specialists and to undergo tests for her very vague complaints. The test results were largely unremarkable, which frustrated her daughters. They complained to the specialists, to the facility, and to me for not solving the mystery of their mother's bouts of illness. The good news, however, was that she recovered just as quickly as she became ill.

In fact she could turn on a dime, so to speak. A good example is the day a reporter from the local newspaper came out unexpectedly to do an article on long-term care at the facility. He arrived on one of those days when Rose had taken to her bed. As soon as she got word from a nurse about the reporter's presence, she leapt up and headed for her closet. Rose had a beautiful wardrobe and a great figure. Even Parkinson's had not managed to obliterate the lingering signs that she had once been regal. Quickly she dressed, made up her face, and hurried down to the activities room. Sure enough, the photographer along for the story snapped her picture, which made the front page a few days later.

Before long, Rose became known as Sonoma's fickle woman. One day she was in bed, demanding to go to the emergency room. The next day she would be the most gracious resident in the facility, helping other residents to the dining room and assisting in their feeding. On her best days, she helped to organize parties and communal arts and crafts projects. Up and down the halls, she would knock on doors, encouraging those who did not often leave their rooms to come out and join in.

How would a normal care team handle Mrs. Jamison?

A normal care team acts as a patient advocate. Team members listen closely to both the resident and his or her family and use the information to help make care-related decisions. They take into account the resident's personal choices and act upon them.

Fortunately for Mrs. Jamison, that description fit the staff members perfectly who happened to work at Sonoma over the first two years of her residency. Initially, she did not leave her room, even for meals. Her Parkinson's disease had advanced enough to give her trouble chewing and swallowing, and she needed extra time to eat. The social worker at the time suggested that her family bring in a small refrigerator. That way, Mrs. Jamison could eat part of her meal in the dining room and take leftovers to her room to eat later. The new plan worked well. In the dining room, Mrs. Jamison began to get acquainted with her fellow residents.

The nursing staff, meanwhile, expressed concern about her physical complaints. Each care conference that the staff held featured new issues to be addressed. Mrs. Jamison had unexplained abdominal pain, unexplained headaches, and unexplained episodes of lethargy. I continued to see her frequently, ordered new tests, and sent her to specialists. Although none of the tests produced a new diagnosis, the staff and I continued to work with consultants and to read the literature for new, untested explanations for Rose's complaints.

Despite our best efforts, the staff and I did grow resigned to what had become routine. Mrs. Jamison waxed and waned, taking to her bed and then resuming her normal activities, with no active treatment or intervention. What looked like a bizarre if benign lifestyle actually was taking its toll, however. An incremental decline was occurring. Every time she took to her bed, Mrs. Jamison lost a little bit more of her gusto. Apparently, her ceaseless cycle was as wearying for her as it was for everyone else.

Her decline was something that Jennifer, one of the certified nursing assistants, was the first to notice and to begin to study. She and Rose had grown close over the months. On afternoons when Rose was indisposed, Jennifer would linger with her over a daytime soap on television and admire her freshly painted nails. From her closet, Rose let Jenny select a silk dress to wear to her daughter's high school graduation.

One day Jennifer came up and spoke to me.

"Have you ever noticed," she asked me, "how Mrs. Jamison seems to get sick whenever her daughters don't come to see her?"

Both daughters had high-powered careers, which led them to travel frequently. That I knew. Often enough, one or both of them were out of town for a week or two at a time. Yet putting two and two together, as Jennifer had done, had not occurred to me. I was too busy searching for a physical cause for Rose's illness.

I shared Jennifer's observation with the nursing staff and other personnel. The pattern did seem to be there, the rest of the team agreed. Whenever she had an appointment with a specialist or went for a test at the emergency room, Mrs. Jamison was sure to spend time with one or both of her daughters. She would also get a change of scenery, something she longed for, according to a number of the nurses.

The care team scheduled a conference with the Jamison family. The social worker, the facility administrator, the director of nursing, and I attended.

"Your mom's physical complaints still lack a diagnosis, despite years of testing," I began.

"Yet she really perks up when you come to see her," Jennifer said.

"In fact, the rest of the staff have noticed a pattern," the director of nursing confirmed.

The two daughters seemed open to the suggestion that some of their mother's physical complaints might be due to depression and fear, as well as a lack of frequent contact with her family.

"Mother was really sad to leave," Julie told us. She was the older girl whose home Rose had lived in just before she came to Sonoma Ranch. "We made the decision together, but, to tell you the truth, she never wanted to live in an institution. She was a good sport—because she knew I didn't have the time or the energy to have her with me at home." Her words came tumbling out, blurted like a confession.

"I think she felt abandoned by us," Emma said. "So of course I feel guilty." She bit her lip. "It makes my visits to see her here very hard."

"She loves you a lot, though," Jennifer said. "I tell her she has more people in her life than ever, but she says she is lonely without you, her girls."

"She can be really good at trying to overcome her feelings," the social worker explained. "Sometimes she does that by being generous toward the other residents. At other times, she masks her depression through her physical complaints."

The conference between the care team members and Rose's daughters led to further thought and further conversation. Not long after our initial meeting, we were able to gather again and develop a plan of action. Julie would visit their mother every Tuesday. Emma would come every Saturday. They also agreed to cover for each other when away on travel, and they got their husbands to take their mother-in-law out occasionally for dinner or a movie.

Within a short time, the results of this plan were as dramatic as Mrs. Jamison herself. Her physical complaints resolved to a significant degree. If she remained a moody person, her ups and downs were less steep. Far more consistent in her behavior and actions, she developed closer bonds with other residents. As for the staff, they took her occasional physical complaints seriously again.

Several months after our care team conference with her family, Mrs. Jamison became the chair of the Sonoma Ranch resident counsel and grew quite involved in organizing senior activities across several long-term facilities.

One weekend, Julie called to ask her to dinner. Rose declined: She had an organizational meeting for the Senior's Ball.

Mrs. Jamison's eventual adjustment to long-term care stemmed from cooperation between a functional care team and a functional family. Together we were able to identify her needs and work cooperatively to satisfy them.

About a year after this resolution, changes took place in the staff at Sonoma. Excellent staff left the facility, and new staff came on in nursing and administration. The changes upset Mrs. Jamison's equilibrium. Her moodiness was something that she never overcame entirely. In fact, the old care team had learned to accommodate her moods, something the new staff, of course, had yet to understand. As for Rose, she was keenly aware of what she termed "blunders" by the "clumsy" newcomers.

A worse blow came when Rose's pet nursing assistant left Sonoma Ranch to help run her family's horse farm. The nursing assistant who replaced Jennifer was not to Mrs. Jamison's liking. She grew needier and more demanding. Expenditure of extra nursing time did not seem to solve her problems. When Rose was not happy, neither was her family. Nowadays when they came in for their weekly visits, Julie and Emma spent far less time chatting with their mother and much more time quizzing the nursing staff, the administrative staff, and me.

How would a bickering care team handle Mrs. Jamison?

A bickering (dysfunctional) care team exists when multiple team members have varying opinions on care. Care team members often give each other mixed or conflicting information, which in turn is often misinterpreted and disjointed when relayed to the resident and the family. Nothing is consistent, which leads to confusion, anger, and frustration. A dysfunctional care team feeds off a person like Mrs. Jamison, and a dysfunctional care team is just what we had become during this period of high staff turnover at Sonoma Ranch.

Team members disagreed on how they saw Mrs. Jamison. The new day nurse thought she was very ill. She called me with Rose's every concern. The new night nurse, on the other hand, thought that Mrs. Jamieson was a faker and refused to give her any of her as-needed medications (such as to ease pain) when she asked for them.

Meanwhile, Mary Turnbull, the housekeeper, who came into Mrs. Jamison's room every day to clean, had become friendly with the Jamison daughters. Perhaps the friendship bloomed because Mary's was one of the few faces the two women still recognized on their mother's floor. In any event, Mary told them of a new drug advertised on television that had worked wonders on her ailing brother-in-law. She must have been persuasive, because the Jamison women went immediately to see Marielle Simpson, the facility administrator, to insist that their mother be put on this medication.

Apparently, the Jamisons had not asked Mary Turnbull exactly what the drug was for or what it was supposed to do. Apparently, Marielle Simpson did not inquire about it either. The "source" of this medical tip went unmentioned.

Not in a position to order medications, Marielle told the women to take their request to me. Like any good administrator, Marielle knew how to please. As she let me know later, "I told them that I was sure you would prescribe any new medicine that would benefit their mother."

Julie called me that same afternoon. We arranged a meeting several days later in the facility to discuss treatment options.

In the interim, Mrs. Jamison complained of severe abdominal pain. I ordered several tests that were performed that same day. The test results came back negative, but Mrs. Jamison did not improve. Julie and Emma arrived to take her to the emergency room, where a physician diagnosed possible gallstones, and then brought her back to Sonoma Ranch.

The next day I entered the facility conference room for my scheduled appointment with the Jamison daughters. Twenty minutes after they had failed to show up, I went down to their mother's room. She was having one of her good days.

"Why don't we follow up on the ER suggestion that your pain might come from gallstones?" I suggested to her. "You could see a specialist for further evaluation and possible surgery."

"I'd like that," she agreed.

I left her with a smile on her face. "At last, I have a 'real' diagnosis," she told me.

Several hours later a received a call from Nancy Murphy, the nursing supervisor. "I got a call from Julie Jamison this afternoon. She was livid. Why haven't you prescribed the new medicine for her mother?"

"We had an appointment scheduled earlier today," I explained. "I had expected to discuss the possibility then. Only no one showed up. I know nothing about this new medication, other than that it may have helped Mary Turnbull's brother-in-law."

"Perhaps you need to bone up a little, then, on the latest," Nancy replied. I heard the edge in her voice, though I tried to ignore it.

"Look," I said. "It is not at all clear that this medication is even relevant. I have no idea what Mary Turnbull's brother-in-law's health problems are. It's something she saw advertised on TV, for heaven's sake."

"Well, there's more," Nancy continued. "They're furious that you discussed surgery for gallstones."

"Why in the world not?"

"The other daughter—Emma—ran into Alice Hastings, when they brought Mrs. J. back here from the ER."

Alice was a new nurse whom I barely knew.

"She pulled Emma aside to give her the news that her mother would never withstand any type of surgery."

A week later, I went in to see Mrs. Jamison. She look downcast and seemed quite despondent.

"I want to be evaluated for surgery, but I am afraid," she told me.

"You can see a surgeon and at least get an evaluation," I explained.

She shook her head. "No. I've been told that it can't be done."

"I don't see why not," I told her.

Mrs. Jamison remained convinced that the surgery was not possible. Although her pain subsided, she called her daughters frequently to tell them about her "incurable" illness. The newer staff began to think that she was terminally ill and to give her extra attention.

A month or so later, the director of nursing, who was also new to Sonoma, called me after a care team meeting.

"The staff met with the family," she said. "Everyone is in

agreement to put Mrs. Jamison into hospice care. All we need now is your okay."

Not quite everyone. Nancy Murphy, the nursing supervisor, was on vacation.

With a diagnosis like Mrs. Jamison's—possible gallstones and no complications—the answer was clear, though bound to be more grist for our bickering care team.

"I don't think that hospice would be appropriate," I replied.

In the spring, Mrs. Jamison's beloved daughter Julie received a job promotion that transferred her too far away to visit. Daughter Emma, meanwhile, continued to travel frequently. Her visits to her mother dwindled from once a week to once a month.

Mrs. Jamison grew more distant from the other residents. In June, her term ended as the head of the resident council. She refocused on her health and placed more demands on the nurses.

She also developed a startling new habit. She screamed in pain. When staff ran into her room to see what was the matter, she demanded that they call Julie, whose long-distance number she had trouble dialing.

"Nobody is going to call Julie unless you behave," the night nurse scolded. "You're waking up everybody on the floor."

Even Nancy Murphy, who had made special efforts to placate her, lost patience now.

"You need to go to the emergency room when you're in that much pain," she told Rose. "You're making life miserable for the other residents."

"There's no one to take me there," Rose shouted. Then she burst into tears.

The change in Rose precipitated a change in members of the care team, who went from bickering among themselves to threatening the resident and her family.

❧

How would a threatening care team handle Mrs. Jamison?

The threatening care team warns of unpleasant consequences, should a resident or family disagree with the staff's views, or with the care plan or facility policy.

❧

Marielle Simpson, the facility administrator, called Emma and arranged for an emergency conference.

"I know that your mother is sad not to see you and Julie as much as she would like," Marielle began the meeting by saying, "but I'm afraid that she has become a problem resident."

The director of nursing broke in then to provide Emma with the details, ticking them off on her fingers. "She fakes illness for attention, places way too many demands on the staff, and disrupts the lives of the other residents."

"She screams a lot," the nursing assistant added with a nod.

Marielle sighed. "That is a problem," she agreed. "Just the other day, I was giving a family a tour of the facility, which they were considering for their own mother. Well, needless to say, your mother's screaming did not leave a good impression."

The nursing assistant snickered.

Marielle sat up tall. "We run an excellent facility," she said, directing herself to Emma. "Sonoma Ranch is part of a premier corporation with prestigious facilities across the country. I expect residents to be well behaved—I'd even say grateful—for the opportunity to live here. If your mother is not satisfied, she should consider going elsewhere."

"I'd think twice, if I were you," the director of nursing stepped in to say. "I can tell you some real horror stories about the alternatives."

"Rose is certainly free to leave," Marielle went on, "but I'm afraid that we would not be able to take her back, if she changed her mind."

As the meeting ended, Rose's daughter Emma looked pale and shaken. She thanked Marielle for her time and shook her hand. Afterward, she paid a visit to her mother. On her way out, I ran into her in the hall.

"I told Mom to stop complaining," she said.

But Mrs. Jamison did not stop complaining. In fact she became more demanding, not less. Nurses and ancillary staff devoted a large part of their shifts to her anxiety, headaches, and abdominal pain. She would ask for the nursing assistant, the nurse, and the physician all at once. All would be contacted and a variety of opinions and plans of action considered. Care conferences were set up to document various complaints and possible alternative plans. The team developed a care plan to address her "issues." Mrs. Jamison was certainly well cared for on paper, but genuine concern for her had diminished. In turn, the care she received became less attentive. Once again, the care team morphed and took on another mood, as threats gave way to distance and a mountain of paperwork.

How would an absent care team handle Mrs. Jamison?

The absent care team is one that is generally unavailable to residents and their families. Team members are preoccupied with their own interactions and more concerned about managing the facility than with providing care to the residents. Providing care has become an institutional concern, distinct and apart from the welfare of the residents. Little effort is made to to promote well-being on an individual basis.

As time passed, the administrative members of the care team grew restive: Mrs. Jamison's care had become expensive. Her health had not stabilized. She continued to have complaints despite intervention. Her care plan did not look particularly "polished," Marielle, the facility administrator, noted, because there had been no resolution of Rose's problems.

In response, someone on the staff came up with a bright idea: Why not change her diagnosis of "abdominal pain" to "*history* of abdominal pain? If the documentation were changed, the "problem" would be diffused over time and crop up as less of an immediate issue in her chart.

I agreed to sign off on the change. The adjustment was not inaccurate. Though it meant more on paper than it did to Mrs. Jamison, it might placate state inspectors when they came into the facility to review resident care plans.

Mrs. Jamison's health continued to decline. She complained of head pain, but its location and severity varied, depending on who asked. Marielle called me in one day to see if I could handle Mrs. Jamison's situation "more proactively."

Before taking any action, it would be necessary to contact her daughters. The facility required their permission to do new testing and to prescribe new medications. Once reached, they agreed to the proactive approach, which was not surprising. Their acquiescence was long standing. From the outset, Mrs. Jamison's daughters had agreed to poor medical care in the form of excessive tests and medications to appease their mother. Would it not have been more constructive if they had just managed to come and visit Rose more often, instead of taking her to doctors and the emergency room? Perhaps they were afraid to take more responsibility for her welfare. In any case, they left most decisions to their mom and her professional caregivers.

I sent Rose to a psychiatrist, whereupon she received prescriptions for anxiety and depression. She started to see a psychotherapist for counseling sessions. On one occasion, she told the therapist that she was sad.

"Have you ever considered suicide?" the therapist asked.

"I've thought about it," Mrs. Jamison said.

The counselor repeated Rose's response to the director of nursing, whose job it was to call Emma and relay facility policy. Anyone who expressed a suicidal intention was to be admitted to the psychiatric ward of the nearest hospital.

Emma was out of town until Friday, but Sonoma Ranch policies left no leeway to wait until her return. The facility had no choice but to contact the psychiatrist who worked with Sonoma Ranch. Mrs. Jamison was admitted to the hospital.

At no time during this transfer process did any member of the administrative care team inquire further about Mrs. Jamison's suicidal thoughts—if indeed she really had any. Nor did anyone on the administrative team ask how Mrs. Jamison would go about killing herself, assuming that she wanted to. She could not walk, and she had no access to harmful medications or weapons. Such questions were simply not relevant to her care plan or to the facility's administrative policy.

Neither Emma nor I were present at the facility on the day that an ambulance took Rose to the psychiatric ward. She had no idea where she was headed or why, a nursing assistant told me later. "She thought she was going in for another x-ray, poor dear."

Mrs. Jamison spent but a few days at the hospital, just long enough to be observed and tested and then discharged. She returned to Sonoma Ranch more subdued than she had been in quite some time. Her mood change was one that the staff naturally welcomed, especially the newer members. Among them was a nurse, Susan Marshall, who took a fancy to Rose, much as Jennifer, the nursing assistant, had once done. Life grew calmer. Emma was able to visit her mother frequently, and Rose began to take some of her meals in the communal dining room.

At Christmas time, Mrs. Jamison reciprocated the kindness that she had received from Susan and some of the other new staff on her return from the hospital. She had the income to give generous gifts.

The new year, however, brought many changes, including a shift in the care team from absent to passive.

How would a passive care team handle Mrs. Jamison?

The passive care team is a hybrid of the absent and the threatening team. Care team members are difficult to contact. Yet they become irate and threatening about not being informed once they learn of resident and family problems and concerns. Occasionally, they provide intense personal interaction with a few favored residents. Such a team often is composed of a core group of staff whose members have worked at the facility for a long time as well as several satellite groups whose members remain in the facility only for a short time.

In January, Mrs. Jamison lost her favorite nurse when Susan Marshall took extended medical leave for surgery. In her absence, the facility called on an agency to provide a temporary replacement. Then one aide quit, and the new one was indifferent to Mrs. Jamison's charm. The weather was poor, and Emma did not drop by as often as she usually did.

Mrs. Jamison's mood declined. More often than not, she stayed in her room and cried. It was at about this time that the aide who worked the day shift began to observe that Rose was more self-sufficient and cooperative with the aide who worked the night shift. The day aide was put out.

"Why won't you dress yourself in the morning? You put your jammies on at night. You're just lazy, that's all. I'm not going to help you anymore unless you shape up, Mrs. Jamison," the aide threatened.

The nurse filling in for Susan Marshall agreed that Mrs. Jamison was lazy. "She should undergo another psychiatric evaluation," she insisted.

Mrs. Jamison agreed to see the psychiatrist again.

"I don't need to see him," Rose told me flatly. "Be that as it may, what with all the coming and goings around here, it's just as well that I find a friendly ear wherever I can."

The nursing staff awaited the psychiatrist's evaluation, hoping for vindication and proof that Mrs. Jamison was "lazy."

The physician indicated that Rose had mild depression and recommended counseling. He would see her in a month.

Mrs. Jamison developed pain. Multiple tests were done, all of which were normal. She demanded constant attention and nursing care, and reverted to her old cycle.

Relief came in the form of Susan Marshall, who returned from medical leave. Mrs. Jamison was ecstatic to see her. At first, so were the other members of the nursing staff. Their pleasure, however, was short-lived. Susan was not happy. In fact, she was irate.

"Why didn't anybody tell me how bad off Rose is," she demanded to know from her colleagues.

"You weren't here," an aide answered.

"I made it a point to call the facility several times," Susan said. "I expected better than this. I expected to be kept informed about my residents."

Susan's reproaches were not well received.

When she persisted, the rest of the staff began to roll their eyes and shrug.

She called the corporate hot line and complained about the facility.

Naturally her call alarmed Marielle Simpson, the facility administrator. In short order, Susan was assigned to a different wing.

"She was just too involved with Rose," everyone said.

Even after her transfer, Susan continued to visit Mrs. Jamison. The two of them watched television together and, like the former nursing assistant Jennifer, she occasionally borrowed some of Mrs. Jamison's clothes.

Their renewed bond did not last much more than a month. Marielle Simpson fired Susan Marshall for being late to work on one too many occasions. As a terminated staff member, Susan could no longer visit Rose. Facility policy forbade her access to the premises.

Having lost Susan twice, Mrs. Jamison sunk back into what her favorite nurse had called "despondency." Her fickleness was becoming a thing of the past. Her mood no longer swung, weighed down by a steady listlessness.

Further change occurred on a larger scale. A buyout of the corporation that owned Sonoma Ranch caused ripples across its holdings nationwide. Marielle Simpson lost her job.

How would no care team affect Mrs. Jamison?

No care team is the result of transience and turnover. Employees are hired from an outside agency; they may work in the facility only once or twice. Staff turnover, even among administrators and nurses, is high. Communication among care team members is nearly nonexistent.

In an episode reminiscent of what had disrupted Tammy Shest's life, the new administrator would no longer allow residents to keep small refrigerators in their rooms. Legal and safety concerns, he announced, meant that the maintenance staff would remove all small appliances. The new policy had a profound effect on Mrs. Jamison whose Parkinson's disease had made her a slow eater. For years she had taken what she could of her meals in the social atmosphere of the dining room and then finished what remained on her plate back in her room, where a social worker had suggested she install a small refrigerator for any leftovers. With the refrigerator's removal, she gave up on the dining room and opted to snack in her room on convenience foods rather than leave half her food on her dinner plate. The social worker who had suggested a refrigerator for the room no longer worked at Sonoma. She might have coaxed Rose into not worrying about wasting good food, but no one else could.

"I was too well-brought up to do a thing like that," she said.

Her reasoning angered the night nurse.

"Why don't you go to dinner like a normal person," she harangued and then noticed that Mrs. Jamison seemed anxious. One weekend the night nurse apparently had had enough. She persuaded the doctor on call to prescribe a "nerve" pill for this "edgy woman." The doctor prescribed a low-dose medication.

The medication confused Rose. She tried to get to the bathroom on her own and fell. She broke her hip. She was hospitalized, where she developed an infection and remained for some time, often in a state of delirium. Eventually, she recovered enough to return to Sonoma Ranch, where she had good days and bad days.

That summer, a new medical director arrived. There was nothing wrong with the old director, namely, Dr. Josephson. It was just that the new corporate administrator had emphasized how important it was for the facility to increase its profits. Thus the facility administrator felt it necessary to find a medical director with more business sense than Dr. Josephson had, one who could refer more seniors to Sandalwood, the newly named facility.

Mrs. Jamison had come to rely on Dr. Josephson. In the last year, he had replaced me as her personal physician, as I severed ties with the new corporation that had bought Sonoma Ranch. She enjoyed his monthly visits, and I felt I had left her in good hands.

Now that he was gone, only a few staff remained who had known Rose from the beginning.

"Why did he leave?" she would ask.

No one could say.

Rose, being Rose, persisted.

One day she put her question to a nurse from an agency, on assignment for her first and probably last time in the facility. Of course the nurse had no idea who Dr. Josephson was, or why he had left.

"I heard he was arrested and lost his license," someone overheard her say.

Rose grew worried. She heard some of the staff laugh at what the nurse said. She did not know whom to trust.

The new medical director came in shortly after that episode to reassess her state of health. He skimmed through the records. He ordered numerous tests. Mrs. Jamison did not improve. In fact, she became worse. She took to her bed. She summoned Emma.

"As you can see, I'm getting ready to die, dear. Please tell your sister to fly in and see me before it's too late."

Mrs. Jamison did not die, not at that point, although Parkinson's disease had made eating a less than pleasant activity for some time. Her retirement from the dining room had begun to have serious consequences. Her nutrition was now poor, and she ate little, refusing supplements and vitamins.

As the care team absorbed the changes that new corporate management brought, its reconstituted membership turned inward. To survive and adjust, the team focused on the facility itself and its own needs. Vestiges of the absent care team resurrected themselves. Providing care had once again become an institutional concern, distinct and apart from the welfare of the residents.

How did a second encounter with an absent care team affect Mrs. Jamison?

During a team conference, Larry Morris, a dietician, spoke up about Rose. He was one of the very few staff who had known her a long time. "We can't let her die without a care plan," he said.

Larry arranged a conference with Mrs. Jamison and her daughter Emma to discuss her mother's deteriorating diet.

"I will die drinking wine and eating chocolate," Rose announced in her grandest manner.

As a matter of written record, she went against medical advice and refused supplemental feeding and drinks. In that case, hospice was the only option, according to facility policy.

Emma obeyed her mother's wishes and signed her up for hospice. Her diagnosis was end-stage Parkinson's disease and malnutrition.

Larry Morris developed a care plan that read roughly as follows:

The resident continues to refuse medical interventions and is losing weight. She is a hospice resident and in a terminal process. Weight loss is to be expected. Given resident's short life-span expectancy, she may eat as she chooses.

The medical director documented Mrs. Jamison's terminal process and the unavoidability of her weight loss. The nursing staff documented her refusal of interventions.

Rose lasted until the spring when her dutiful daughters arrived with a basket of goodies. Though unable to partake, there at her fingertips were the glass of red wine and the box of dark chocolates, just as she had wanted, at the end of her life.

7

At the Crux of Care — Four Ways to Death

Once a care team becomes an individual's professional family, a system to manage a person's care needs to be selected and applied. Each management system provides a structure to live and work by. Each has the goal of producing a positive outcome. What constitutes a positive outcome (good care), differs, however, for each system, which has its own dominant means to achieve its goal. Four basic models are available for facilities to choose from and rely on in offering resident care.

- The scientific model
- The business model
- The social model
- The ethical model

Each of these management systems is used to find an answer for death, illness, and aging. The scientific—or medical—model offers us a hope for a cure through medical breakthroughs and advanced technology. The business model offers us a lowdown on the statistics—the odds on when and how we will age with all its attendant risks—and then the insurance plans, which we can pay to cover our eventual losses and for our institutional care. Near the end of life, the social—or hospice care—model offers us compassion and comfort, if we can resign ourselves that we are going to die. Ethical management is based on moral principles and values, or a guiding philosophy. Although unaffiliated with religion per se, this model does focus on the spiritual life of the individual. The crux of this approach is personal responsibility. The values identified in the model may lead the user to accept or reject one or more of the other models described above. The goal is to provide care that is deemed ethical by all parties involved.

These first three systems do work well in response to crisis situations: The person who is acutely ill with a myocardial infarction may be saved by the science of medical intervention and care. The young father who dies unexpectedly may benefit his family by having had the business sense to invest in insurance. The elder who develops a terminal cancer may find solace in hospice.

Truth and Science

The Scientific Management System marshals all products of the long-term care professional disciplines—from medical practice to drugs to therapies to nursing to social services and nutrition—and brings them to bear in determining appropriate care and progress for the resident. The resulting care plan is the crux of the scientific model. The model assumes that the resident will agree and act on this "logical" plan. When residents do not agree to the "truth" of such care plans, they or their families must sign a disclaimer. The goal of the Scientific Management System is to defeat death, disability, and illness.

Once a facility adopts the Scientific Management System, each resident must have a care plan, a written document developed by care team members. As the centerpiece of the system, the care plan consists of what the resident should or should not do. It is a list of "problems" as well as their "solutions."

Each plan undergoes an update at least quarterly. Acute Plans of Care (APOC) are developed, should events take place in the interim (before the next quarterly update). Many aspects of aging can prompt the need for a new plan, just as the scientific model seeks to address associated problems. These problems can include pain, depression, weight (gain or loss), falls, skin breakdown, blood pressure, diabetic management, poly-pharmaceutical usage (nine or more medications prescribed), risk-reduction medications, maintenance medications, and the dying process.

Security and Business

The Business Management System aims to obtain a good statistical outcome in terms of financial gains and losses that arise out of long-term care. Good care is simply defined as fewer lawsuits (losses) and the least expensive care for the price paid (gains). The insurance industry is the crux of this system, as it apportions financial accountability and responsibility. The goal is to ensure that the facility is economically profitable. Although the resident is not at the center of this model, quality care need not be excluded.

Insurance analyzes positive and negative factors and assigns a risk for almost any variable imaginable. Business takes these variables and consolidates them into something positive. Originally, insurance protected the individual against catastrophic loss, say, against fire (the loss that insurance came into being to cover).

What used to be an option has now become a requirement: Car owners need insurance to register their vehicles and drive, homeowners need insurance to get a mortgage, patients need insurance to visit doctors, and physicians need insurance to practice their profession.

Sometimes the risk is too high to cover. In a catch-22, government and business require us to be insured, but insurance companies prefer to cover those who do not need coverage (low risk). Although we are forced to acquire insurance, the industry is not forced to take us, even if we are willing to pay a high price in exchange for the high risk. Doctors who take care of elderly people who may die, or pregnant women who may have imperfect children, can be denied insurance, which itself can be catastrophic.

Yet this scenario, too, has altered in recent years. Once insurance became universally required, coverage began to extend to events that do have a high probability of happening. Today few parts of life exist for which we cannot buy protection. Instead of taking preventive measures to protect our health, say, by taking our diabetic medicine or following a proper diet, we can pay for insurance to cover eventual medical treatment. Doctors, in turn, rely on insurance to protect them from their mistakes.

Some individuals who are fortunate enough to have expansive health care coverage will avail themselves of services more frequently than they might otherwise. Insurance becomes a luxury item. Its privileges can be wielded to shift responsibility for health from the individual to the professional. In reality, the professional cannot really take responsibility but only offer options, though such options do shape the decisions that individuals then make.

When it comes to long-term care, the shift in responsibility becomes ever more complex, as it is not just the individual who relies on the professional for advice, but also the family, who renounces responsibility in favor of the professional "family" or care team at the long-term facility. The more individuals are involved, the more complex the dynamics will be.

If insurance constitutes a large pool of money into which individuals and businesses dip, the resident of the long-term care facility is rather like a commodity who is traded based on a risk category. In my experience, it sometimes seems that all human emotion is wrung from the care that residents receive. The business and scientific models have become so sophisticated that it is almost too risky to house residents, given their "quirks." Certainly it is too risky to allow residents to age or to die in long-term care facilities without a care plan. The social model does offer the resident emotional care. However, that care is predicated on the acceptance of one's imminent death. For some conditions, this option is a good one.

Compassion and Society

The Social Management System integrates diverse sources of care—spiritual, familial, and professional—on a comfort, not a curing, basis. The pinnacle of the social model is hospice care. The resident who enters such care is expected to acknowledge the uselessness of a scientific plan, because a cure is not feasible, and he or she has reached a terminal state. Scientific aspects of medicine, such as drugs and tests, are relied on only to comfort the resident. Death has been agreed upon, though the time frame is unclear.

Hospice originated as a grassroots organization to help dying people and their families. It was, and continues to be, a wonderful source of relief and support to dying people and their loved ones. Among the benefits that hospice offers to those with a terminal diagnosis are:

- aggressive management of symptoms, such as pain, anxiety, and restlessness at the end of life;
- social support for the family in terms of spiritual and emotional assistance, as well as medical and respite assistance;
- continuous human contact at the end of life;
- specialized comfort equipment such as an electric bed or oxygen that may be too expensive for the family to afford.

Over time, hospice care has had to evolve to survive. It has done so by capitalizing on the shortcomings of the scientific and business models, neither of which responds well to unpredictability. Thus hospice comes to the rescue and offers a respectable transition from the scientific plan, stymied by the incurable problems of aging. Hospice offers a care plan for death and a way to resolve noncompliance with the proscribed medical regime. In entering hospice care, the resident has resigned to die, reducing the likelihood of a wrongful death lawsuit against the facility and care team. Likewise, hospice offers a "cure" for the business plan. When lawsuits are less of a threat, nonaggressive care can be provided inexpensively and thus ensure profits.

Yet devising such solutions is still not enough. Caring for dying people is simply not sufficiently marketable and profitable. Hospice care has had to continue to struggle for a way to support itself. The longer the patient is enrolled, of course, the larger the profits. Thus a growing trend has been to extend hospice care to people earlier in the dying process. Those who are chronically ill—with dementia, chronic bronchitis, and coronary disease—are often able to qualify. The trend may also benefit family members, as hospice covers some things that traditional insurance will not.

However, enrollment in a hospice is a pivotal step. The resident must agree (on paper) that he or she is dying. I believe that the process is suggestive. Signing on to such a statement can and does alter the resident's ability to heal and affects his or her mental outlook. Agreeing to death means death.

Ethics and Religion

The Ethical Management System offers us acceptance of aging, illness, and death as natural parts of life, which need not be hurried on the one hand, nor denied and defied on the other. Those who espouse this approach use the other systems when necessary but do not artificially place natural aging in the crisis domain. Why do we not seek this last model more often? Is it because we resist its conclusions? Would we rather not accept aging, illness, and death as natural and inevitable?

Choosing to follow an ethical model in long-term care tends to fly in the face of values that dominate our culture today. Among other things, we are risk-averse and therefore more passive. Witness our tendency to rely heavily on professionals for advice and to make our decisions for us, whereas, under the Ethical Management System, the well-being and security of the resident are thought of first and foremost in terms that are private and individual. Decision making is a matter of personal responsibility, independent of outside "forces" such as insurance companies and regulators. Our fear of the risks involved in taking personal responsibility means we rely more than ever on outside recognition and affirmation in order for our decisions to seem real at all, let alone virtuous.

Although we are afraid of the risks involved in responsibility, we are eager to brandish our values in a general way. If ethics cannot be bought and sold, our visible embrace of them can be. As a profit-driven society, we are encouraged to profess our outlooks and values as though they were items to be marketed. We cannot wait for someone to get to know us. Instead we must wear a t-shirt or a button to instantly advertise what we believe and what we value. Of course, the signals we send are no real indication of how we will actually behave. The bumper sticker on a car that says "Trust in God" does not necessarily mean that the driver really does.

Similarly, the preaching of beliefs has become a marketing tool to urge us to purchase a "packaged deal" of morality and salvation. Going through the motions of an organized religious service once a week may make us feel more secure, but it does not necessarily signify a life guided by ethical principle. At the end of the day, our deeds and the choices that preceded them reveal our real moral status. All around us, meanwhile, we constantly hear someone referred to as a "person of faith." To question such a label implies hostility. "Don't question my heart," we are often told, even by our country's President. Our hearts are too private to know firsthand, it would seem. We must take each other on faith.

Codes of Kindness

Not so in the nursing home, however, where any good deed that is not well documented is easily dismissed. Even more troublesome, any act that goes unrecorded may well be viewed as sneaky and underhanded no matter how virtuous. Without the bureaucratic hand of the administrator to codify each random act of kindness as a type of caregiving officially recognized by the state, virtue remains suspect. Indeed the resident who wrote the poem that inspired me to write this book had it right: We have arrived at the point in long-term care where God, too, needs a risk manager to protect and promote ethics.

Several times in my career, I have interviewed for a position as a medical director of a facility. The most common questions that I was asked during the interview were:

- What hospital system are you associated with (marketing or business)?
- Can you provide patient referrals?
- How do you document your visits? Do you rely on care plans and evaluate key issues such as weight loss and skin problems?
- What else can you offer the facility? Do you feel comfortable speaking on the lecture circuit or attending dinners or other events, which the facility sponsors to promote the facility?

Rarely have I been asked to demonstrate that I practice good medicine or that I care about resident patients and their families. I do not recall ever being asked to discuss any clinical issues or to talk about my philosophy of care.

Long-term health care facilities definitely do need to use scientific, business, and social models to operate. Ethics, however, remain an afterthought. As current thinking has it, once we embrace the scientific, business, or social model, ethics will follow naturally. They do not.

8

The Enigma of the Care Plan

The most important part of care can be the care plan itself. Sadly, I have seen many instances of good care plans that document what is actually substandard care. Conversely, I have seen many instances of good care underwritten by poor plans. Unfortunately, bad care is not penalized to the same degree as a bad plan. Care plan assumptions include the following:

- For every treatment, there must be a diagnosis. For every diagnosis, there must be a treatment. (There is a problem that must be addressed.)
- What is documented is the truth.
- What is not documented has not happened.
- Only diagnoses that can be verified by direct testing can be used to establish an illness; negative tests mean no illness exists, at least not on paper.

Intended to ensure good residential care, in practice, the care plan has become a mechanical exercise that can do more harm than good. Widely embraced, it has become a quality indicator for the government (state and federal regulators) to judge long-term care facilities. State surveys often have an unofficial theme, which care plans are expected to reflect. If the government inspectors do not like a given care plan, a POC (plan of correction) must be developed and a re-inspection occurs. Lack of compliance can result in fines. Thus the care plan has become a document to prove that long-term facilities have done no wrong.

Doctors likewise turn to the care plan to substantiate lack of mistakes. It is our insurance against governmental sanctions, angry families, and frivolous lawsuits. Dangerously, we can become more concerned about how each care plan reads on paper than how the corresponding resident appears in person. Also frightening is that we have begun to believe in paper "plans" more than in hands-on attention. Diagnoses and individual risk factors are examined on paper—but not necessarily with regard to the resident. A care plan can be developed by reviewing a resident's chart and without actually physically evaluating him or her. Such documentation can qualify as direct patient care.

Medicating Age

The nursing home pharmacy plays a major role in residential care plans. Drug reviews are conducted every month, though again it is the chart that is reviewed, not the resident. Commonly prescribed medications include drugs for cholesterol, depression, stroke prevention, gastric reflux, and dementia, to name a few. They can be prescribed for those who have no diagnosis for these conditions other than their age. In fact, this type of prescribing has become so rampant over the past several years that it has become standard care.

High cholesterol, diabetes, and hypertension affect many people and effective treatment with drugs does extend lives. Medicating related symptoms among the "captive audience" of elderly people in long-term care means that more drugs can be sold, and the profit is greater. This is not necessarily a bad thing, as it provides money for further funding of important drugs and treatments. Research on drugs can be very expensive. Developing drugs that help only a few is not realistic. All the same, medicating residents who have little or nothing to gain has become the norm.

Furthermore, not prescribing these "proactive" drugs has become a liability and is viewed as a contradiction of the care plan. Residents with osteoporosis, and those who are at risk for cerebral vascular accident or stroke or heart attack, are expected to be put on "risk-reduction" medications. If they are not, their care plans are flagged by state and federal regulators. Medications that reduce disease or morbidity are beside the point. Risk reduction trumps all.

Some aspects of the care plan address problems related to aging and illness that can be dealt with appropriately through medical interventions. In other respects, however, the care plan attempts to medicalize what is perfectly normal and natural. It is problematic, then, to be required to document interventions into what is a normal process. The care plan itself can be contradictory. I am asked to treat pain, but pain medications can cause falls. I must not put a resident on too many medications, but the resident must be on all medications appropriate to his or her diagnoses. In the end, I am usually forced to resolve such contradictions myself.

Most ironic, is the last "problem" on my care plan list—death. Can a person die without a care plan? As a general rule, no. Administrators and professionals tend to refuse to let a resident die in their facilities without such a plan. Either I send the dying resident to the emergency room, or I must persuade him or her to agree to hospice care.

Residents need treatment of curable medical illnesses, prevention of the progression of diseases (if possible), and alleviation of symptoms if a cure is not possible. A care plan may help to accomplish these objectives, as long as the resident's interests are not subordinate to the care team's own need to ensure that the facility looks good to state inspectors. Two actual, though not unusual, incidents show how a care plan can work in practice. Whether the incident happens in a facility or at home can make a sharp difference.

Arlene Glassman came to the Sweet Penny Tree nursing facility when she was eighty-three. She had few medical problems. Her decline was due simply to wear-and-tear aging. If Mrs. Glassman's body was failing her, her mind was clear. It was not unusual for her to leave the premises and go off somewhere with her children.

Catching a Cold

At her daughter's home one weekend, Arlene came down with a cold. She wanted some over-the-counter medications to relieve her symptoms. Obligingly, her daughter went up to the local pharmacy and brought back a decongestant, some cough medicine, and an analgesic. Mrs. Glassman took the medicines as needed. She improved without consequence after a week.

Two months later, Arlene again came down with a cold. This time she was at Sweet Penny Tree, where, at about ten a.m. on a Saturday morning, Mrs. Glassman first mentioned to the nurse on duty that she had a cold. The nurse looked at her orders and saw that she had none for as-needed medications.

"I'll have to call the doctor to get an order," she told Arlene.

Several hours passed. Mrs. Glassman asked the nurse again for some cough medicine.

"I'm sorry," the nurse told her. "I got busy and didn't get a chance to call the doctor." A shift change was then in process. "I'll let the incoming nurse know."

Again, several hours passed. When Mrs. Glassman mentioned cough medicine to the new nurse on duty, she was not receptive. "It is eight p.m. on a Saturday," she said, "and I am not going to call a doctor for cough medicine. You will just have to wait until the morning."

At nine p.m., Mrs. Glassman's daughter arrived to visit and to bring her mother some cough medicine. The nurse came in and saw Arlene swallow a spoonful. She removed the bottle from Arlene's nightstand.

"Not only is this patient not permitted to keep medicines in her room," she informed Mrs. Glassman's daughter, "she has no physician order for cough syrup."

At this point, Mrs. Glassman and her daughter became angry. They demanded that the physician be called.

The nurse shook her head. "First, I have to call my supervisor about the unauthorized use of cough medicine."

The supervisor called the director of nursing at home, who, in turn, called the administrator. In the interim, the physician on call happened to phone in regarding another resident. One of the nurses, who liked Arlene, picked up the phone and asked him for an order for cough syrup.

This time, Mrs. Glassman got off with a warning against her "clandestine" use of a tablespoon of cough medicine.

Mrs. Glassman slept through the night. In the morning, she felt a bit congested, and her muscles ached. She asked for an over-the-counter analgesic and a decongestant. The morning nurse checked her orders.

"I'm sorry, but I have no orders for these medications, though I see you just received one for cough medicine. I'll call to see if you can have the others."

"May I have some more cough medicine, then, please?"

"I'm afraid not," the nurse said. "The doctor's order says every six hours. You'll have to wait a bit."

Later that morning, Mrs. Glassman's son came to pick her up to take her out for lunch.

"Mrs. Glassman is ill," the nurse informed him. "In my judgment, she should not go out."

"It's only a head cold," the son said. "She just needs a decongestant."

The nurse said nothing but gave him a long, disapproving stare.

"Look," the son explained to her, "I am going to take her out for a nice lunch, and first we'll stop at the drug store."

"I can call a physician," the nurse offered.

"That's not necessary," he insisted. "We don't need a doctor for such a mundane issue. I'm going out with Mom as planned."

"Please don't leave until the physician is called," the nurse responded. "Otherwise, you will be leaving against medical advice, which raises insurance and payment issues."

It would also mean that, if the facility so chose, it would not have to take Arlene back as a resident.

The son waited while the nurse called the doctor. Luckily, the one on call that day knew Mrs. Glassman. He ordered the appropriate medications and issued a pass so that she could lunch with her son.

Taking a Fall

Gilbert Pollick, a seventy-year-old with chronic mental illness, had lived in long-term care for many years. His one excursion occurred at Christmas, when he visited his son's home to celebrate the season. During the course of festivities one year, Gilbert tripped over a gift box and fell on the carpet.

"I'm okay," he told his son and picked himself up off the floor with no problem.

At dinner, he mentioned a bit of hip pain, but he waved off his son's question as to whether he should seek medical help. They played cards in front of the fireplace and then went to bed. In the morning over breakfast, Gilbert said that he felt just fine. His son drove him back to the facility.

I did not learn of Gilbert's fall at his son's home until the following year when Gilbert made an offhand remark as he waited for his son to pick him up on Christmas Eve.

"I hope Lenny got rid of that lousy carpet. I tripped on the damn thing the last time."

The following spring, Gilbert slipped on the way back to his room from the facility dining room. Several of the staff witnessed the fall in the hallway.

"Why don't you get into bed, Gilbert?" one of them suggested.

"I don't need to do that," he said.

"You heard what we said. Go to bed."

Shortly after Gilbert complied, the floor nurse came in and did an assessment. She found nothing wrong. A little while later, the nursing supervisor assessed him as well and reported that he appeared unharmed by the fall. Nonetheless, protocol required the floor nurse to file an incident report, and to schedule Mr. Pollick to receive hourly checks over the next twenty-four-hour period. After the nurse finished the incident report, she faxed it to the facility's law firm in accordance with facility house policy on risk management. As Mr. Pollick's physician, I also was notified of the fall.

For the rest of the day, Mr. Pollick was confined to bed. He was not allowed to go outside to smoke. The restrictions, especially on his smoking, made him angry. During one of his hourly checks, a nurse asked if he was experiencing any pain.

"Well, I do have a little hip pain," Gilbert responded.

The nurse called me, and I ordered a hip x-ray. Again, Gilbert was told to stay in bed until the x-ray results were reported. The x-rays turned up normal, and at last Gilbert was permitted to return to his ordinary activities.

A few weeks later, the state surveyors arrived at the facility. In the course of their review, they found fault with Gilbert's chart with respect to his fall; some of the nursing notes were incomplete.

The surveyors questioned Gilbert directly about the fall.

As Gilbert told me later, he did not really remember much about the events surrounding his fall. However, he did not want to appear stupid. He also wanted to satisfy the surveyors, who seemed eager to hear what he had to say. So he confabulated a story. Some of what he said was true; some was not.

After Gilbert finished his story, it was no longer possible for anyone to sort truth from fiction.One clear-cut question that did remain was whether his hip was x-rayed in a timely manner. Luckily, the order for the x-ray had been documented thoroughly, and the x-ray itself was available immediately. The surveyors were satisfied with its timeliness, and they closed the case, although they did issue the facility a minor citation for improper nursing documentation that did not result in harm to the resident.

A year passed. During an internal audit, Gilbert's chart again underwent review. An entry in the nursing notes indicated that, four months after his fall (and after the state surveyors had reviewed the chart), Gilbert complained of hip pain on the same side of his body on which he had taken his fall.

The internal auditor noted the absence of any documentation to show that his complaint received any follow-up. In fact, Gilbert had voiced no further complaints about hip pain until the aforementioned four months had passed, and the nurse made her note. Still, the internal auditor advised the director of nursing to counsel the nurse on her "error."

9

Gilbert and Grace — Care Gets Manipulated

It is easy enough to see how the different operational models and systems described in the previous chapters affect and shape lives. Take once again Gilbert Pollick as an example. At seventy, Gilbert already had been in the nursing facility for several years when I began to take care of him. Although blessed with few physical problems, he had a long history of chronic mental illness and spent much of his life in psychiatric hospitals. He did have a family, including a son, but they remained only marginally involved in Gilbert's life.

A Lone Worrier

Poor insight, delusions, and paranoia all kept Mr. Pollick from functioning independently. He retained the energy and physical coordination to bathe himself but did not know when to do so. His obsessions and paranoia overwhelmed his physical capacity to take care of day-to-day activities. Instead he used his energy to pace the floors, worrying and fearing that he was ill. Every week when I visited him, he begged me to help him. Whenever he really was ill, however, he refused my care.

Gilbert lived on the behavioral unit, a special place in nursing homes set aside for psychiatric patients. Ideally, such psychiatric units do not house the chronically ill nor residents with dementia, but that is not always the case. In Gilbert's case, the unit included elders with dementia and behavioral problems, young people with traumatic brain injury and impulsive behaviors, as well as chronically ill ex-convicts who had no place to live after parole or discharge.

Gilbert was judged to be annoying but harmless by other residents and care team members alike. If we staff members tended to avoid him, it was largely out of embarrassment, as there was not much that we could do for him, though we were loathe to admit as much. Gilbert was a loner. He would participate in group activities, but would not interact.

Gilbert—The Scientific Model

From the vantage point of the Scientific Management System, Gilbert was an unusual resident. Because of his chronic mental illness, he entered long-term care five years shy of the medically categorized "young-old" age range (seventy-five to eighty-five). He was in the "system" so long that he "aged" into it.

A year after he became my patient, Gilbert began to complain of insomnia. He told me that he had not slept in three days; he told the day nurse that he had not slept in four. The night nurse stated that he slept through the night, but she did not document her observation. In response to Gilbert's complaint, the day shift supervisor instituted an acute plan of care. An APOC requires documentation of the resident's status on every shift for two weeks or until the problem is resolved.

The day shift supervisor called me for medical intervention. In response, I ordered a mild sleeping pill for a limited period of time. Gilbert continued to complain. I ordered another medication. Gilbert continued to complain. I increased his medications. He began dozing off during the day and was counseled to try and stay awake so that he would not have trouble sleeping at night.

The two-week APOC came to an end, but Gilbert's complaint of insomnia continued. The more interventions we instituted, the more needy and demanding he became. A psychiatrist was called in to document both Gilbert's compulsive behavior and his sleeping habits. The psychiatrist tried a new medication. There was no change in Gilbert's condition. The next week the psychiatrist wrote that Gilbert's obsessive mental disorder was causing him to complain of insomnia. Observation proved that he did, in fact, sleep through each night. No treatment was indicated for insomnia. We would treat his mental illness instead. Though Gilbert was no longer diagnosed as an insomniac, his records would continue to show a history of insomnia. At least he did not need a related care plan.

Another year passed. Gilbert began to complain of insomnia again. The staff called me in, and I prescribed a mild sleeping agent, which I kept him on, as the treatment seemed to be effective. No care plan was developed, and the care team agreed that this problem had been addressed in the past and did not need further investigation.

A week later, Gilbert had a new complaint; actually two. He complained of pain and depression. The nursing staff and I evaluated him regarding each problem. Nothing dramatic was noted. Simple testing and interventions were developed into a care plan.

Gilbert continued to complain. In fact, he needed to speak to someone almost constantly. If he was not talking to the nurse, he was talking to the nursing assistant, or the social worker, or the housekeeper, or the phone operator. He did not talk to other residents, however, or engage in small talk or ordinary conversation. He seemed able to talk only about his ill health. At this point, most caregivers avoided Gilbert—he was so anxious to talk but had so little to say.

An acute care plan was formulated for his pain. Gilbert was placed on a variety of pain medications. He underwent an MRI of his bones and a CT scan of his organs. His pain varied in location and in intensity from day to day. He was sent to an orthopedic specialist as well as to a gastroenterologist for more complex testing. No new diagnoses were found. His pain was stabilized after a month or so with an arthritic pill that he took daily, as well as a stronger pain medication that he took on occasion.

Another APOC was developed for his depression, though Gilbert gave no reason for depression. What remained clear and unvarying was his chronic mental illness—schizophrenia and a personality disorder. Again the psychiatrist evaluated him, and several medications were adjusted as well as a new one added. Gilbert was not considered a candidate for counseling, as his insight was too poor. This lack of insight was not substantiated and may or may not have been the case in reality. On paper, however, it was documented fact.

A pharmacy review indicated that Gilbert was at risk for a stroke, as he had a history of high blood pressure. It was also noted that he might benefit from lipid-lowering therapy. He was at risk for falls and might have osteoporosis. The review was silent as to how lifestyle changes might make a difference, say, if Gilbert were to eat a healthier diet and exercise, not to mention were he to quit smoking. Labs were ordered; they were discussed with Gilbert and his guardian. Treatments for possible diseases in the future were instituted. He was placed on a medicine for elevated lipids and two more medications—one for possible osteoporosis (and possible fracture if he did have osteoporosis) and another for a possible stroke (given his risk factors).

Gilbert experienced some side effects from his risk-reduction medications. I placed him on two more medications—one for constipation and one for dizziness. He also complained of acid-reflux and heartburn. I placed him on a stomach medication (a maintenance medication).

I received another pharmacy review. Gilbert's medications had expanded from five to seventeen once the various care plans were instituted.

Before Care Plans (Five)

- Three psychiatric medications (used long term and stabilized)
- Two medications for high blood pressure

After Care Plans (Twelve)

- Sleep medication—one new medication spurred by the initial care plan
- Pain medications—two
- Depression—one new medication added
- "Risk-reduction" medications—four
- Treatment of side effects from risk-reduction medications—three
- Maintenance medication—one (for stomach upsets and heartburn)

Being on more than nine medications had triggered a screen for improper practice of medicine. Furthermore, Mr. Pollick had been taking his medications for insomnia and those related to his psychiatric problems for quite some time. I was asked to document why a dosage reduction had not been tried. State law and long-term care facility policy required that dosage reduction be attempted six months after the current dosage had been prescribed, unless there was a contraindication.

I justified Gilbert's medications by citing his complaints and the various care plans that had been developed, including the recommendations from the pharmacy. All care team members were satisfied with my rationale and with my documentation. Gilbert, however, continued to complain.

Gilbert—The Business Model

Despite his high-maintenance status from a medical management point of view, Gilbert was a desirable resident from the standpoint of business. He had a payer source. He had insurance that covered his physician bills, most medications, most laboratory tests, as well as his room and board. He received a small disability payment, which he turned over to the facility. The administrative office paid his bills and returned whatever money was left. Everyone was happy with the situation. The facility was guaranteed payments, and Gilbert had some spending money.

From a medical standpoint, Gilbert was still young. Statistically, he could live for many years (twenty or more) and remain a constant source of income. Not only statistically young, he appeared at low risk for chronic disease. At that point at least, he required few expensive treatments. His disability payment would cover any treatment that he might later receive in excess of what his insurance would pay.

Also reassuring in terms of legal risks (losses), was his estrangement from the few family members he had left, who might have found a reason to bring a lawsuit or a complaint to the state. Though Gilbert was a complainer, he never asked to go to another facility or home. His annual visit to his son at Christmas was all the family contact that he maintained.

Gilbert had a case manager. She maintained a good caseload of residents, and she made referrals to attract new residents and thus new income (gains) to the facility. As far as she and the facility administrator were concerned, Gilbert was a "model" resident. The facility's goal was to keep him as long as his status did not change.

Gilbert—The Social Model

Gilbert developed an unusual lesion on his head. It grew larger and larger almost daily. He began to pick at it, and it began to bleed. Though very concerned about it, he refused to go to a dermatologist until the lesion had grown across his forehead. Finally, he agreed to an evaluation. An appointment was scheduled with a dermatologist. Gilbert refused to go on the scheduled day, and the appointment was rescheduled.

Eventually he did manage to visit the dermatologist accompanied by one of the staff members whom he trusted somewhat. The dermatologist told Gilbert that a specialized surgeon needed to perform a biopsy. Gilbert agreed to have this procedure done, although he was quite anxious. Both he and the staff asked me to prescribe a sedating medication that he could take beforehand. Though I did prescribe the sedative, he arrived at the surgeon's office so agitated and combative that only a small sample of the tissue could be removed.

A week or so later, the results came back. Most likely, he had some type of malignancy, but the tissue types were mixed (some appeared very malignant; others less so) and more tissue was needed to make a definite diagnosis. Obviously, no treatment could begin until the surgeon knew with certainty what he would be treating.

Gilbert was traumatized. He refused to go back to the surgeon. Usually so eager to flag down staff in the halls, he took to his room. There he stayed, coming out only for a few meals and to smoke his pack of cigarettes. For better or for worse, the staff did not coax him out of seclusion. People preferred Gilbert the Hermit to Gilbert the Nag.

The lesion on his head continued to expand. He could no longer eat with the other residents as the sore bled spontaneously. At about this time, the state surveyors were expected to arrive to inspect the facility. The care team insisted on a management plan for Gilbert. He looked bad. Surely his appearance would raise a "red flag." His chart would be reviewed. A care conference was scheduled. Gilbert was given the options of further treatment or, perhaps, hospice.

Gilbert agreed to meet with hospice care personnel. After much discussion, he enrolled in the program. The application of the social model to Gilbert's case was probably not appropriate. In fact, he had no terminal diagnosis but only one for an undifferentiated cancer, which remained unproven. A cure might have been available for whatever ailed him, only he had forfeited treatment out of fear. As it was, he did not benefit from any of the services that hospice can offer—pain management, special equipment not usually covered by insurance, and emotional and spiritual support.

The LTC facility did not benefit either, at least not economically (business model), because Gilbert's payer source changed. However, it did benefit administratively as Gilbert's care plans grew in detail and appeared more complete (scientific model) as a result of the change in status. The good news was that Gilbert was now happy once he entered hospice. No longer did anyone pester him to make an appointment for an evaluation. Now he could do as he pleased.

A few months went by. Gilbert's lesion actually shrunk a bit. He had no other problems. One evening he developed chest pain for which the doctor on call ordered a palliative medication. Over the weekend he developed shortness of breath and asked to go to the hospital. The nurse on duty did not want to call the doctor, as Gilbert was "hospice." As he grew more ill, however, she relented, and Gilbert was transferred to the ER. There he was diagnosed as having had a heart attack a few days before. While Gilbert was in the hospital recovering from his heart attack, a biopsy was done on his forehead. The lesion was found to be a relatively benign and curable form of skin cancer.

Gilbert—The Ethical Model

From an ethical standpoint, the facility needed to provide good care to Gilbert regardless of costs or facility politics and dynamics. He had a right to have his symptoms and his complaints addressed. As his symptoms were mental rather than physical, counseling and other psychotherapeutic options and plans might have been pursued more aggressively than they were.

Before he entered the hospice program, Gilbert had a right to seek treatment. His refusal to do so was questioned periodically in a nonthreatening way, which is precisely as it should have been from an ethical standpoint. For Gilbert also had the right to refuse treatment. He had no obligation to agree to hospice care just to tweak his care plans.

Gilbert had the right to move to a less restrictive environment, were he capable of doing so. In an ideal world, perhaps he could have become a resident of a group home eventually. Once again from a business standpoint, however, it benefited the facility to keep Mr. Pollick right where he was before he opted for hospice, that is, on the behavioral unit of long-term care, where his consistent income was a boon to the facility.

Grace Denied

The case of Graciella Comas-Diaz shows how a very different sort of patient can fare under each of the four models for long-term care. An eighty-year-old woman with many physical problems—diabetes and a history of strokes and heart problems—Grace arrived at the long-term facility in a fairly advanced stage of dementia. Largely immobile and wheelchair-bound, she came to the facility because she could not live alone. Nor could her two middle-aged daughters care for her. The demands of their respective careers and families made it close to impossible for either of them to offer the kind of round-the-clock care that their mother needed.

It is not unusual for people with advanced dementia to spit out medicines and to fight activities such as bathing and feeding. In Grace's case, she feared her own reflection. If she saw herself in the mirror that hung in the room that she shared with Hope Brown, she would scream. Hope quickly came up with the solution and hung pillow cases over the offending glass. Grace did not like her diapers. She would pull them apart and eat the stuffing. Again, Hope arrived at a solution. It was for her roommate, Grace, that she designed the one-piece outfits with the zippers up the back. Once Grace could no longer pull at her diapers, she grew calm and appeared to forget about them.

In most respects, however, Mrs. Comas-Diaz was a model patient. Far from exhibiting aggressive behavior, she readily complied with her day-to-day care and smiled at her caregivers, even if she did not recognize them. She evoked their sympathy. Sometimes she even fed herself.

Grace—The Scientific Model

From the standpoint of scientific management, Grace was not a desirable resident, given her age and several, serious medical problems. She did not understand questions posed to her. She was incontinent and unable to dress or to wash herself. The scientific model could at least address her diabetes, a condition well controlled with oral medications. The stroke that she suffered several years ago, and from which she had recovered only somewhat, was not so easily managed, however. From the scientific standpoint, realistic goals were to maintain functional status, such as her ability to walk and feed herself occasionally, as well as to prevent further damage from her diabetes, such as infection and skin breakdown.

The first problem Grace encountered when she entered the facility had to do with communication. Her speech was garbled, and she had a limited vocabulary. Her hearing was poor, and she did not comprehend what was said to her. I and the other caregivers had trouble understanding her.

In due course, the care team decided that Grace might be having pain that she was unable to express. A care plan was developed. A scheduled pain pill was given to her before her physical therapy and before bed. A pain medication also was ordered, "as needed," which the nurses could give at their discretion.

She seemed to have increased trouble walking. She was seen by a physical therapist but was not able to carry out her treatment plan with any real success. She was also restless and was having trouble sleeping.

Grace fell one day trying to get out of bed. I was notified, as was her family. An incident report was filed, and an acute plan of care was developed. The incident received attention during the next Falls Committee meeting. Appropriate interventions were put in place. Grace was given a low bed and an alarm system that she could use to signal a problem. She underwent a battery of laboratory tests.

She had another fall and was flagged as "at risk." Her falls had caused her pain. Yet the very medications prescribed to alleviate her discomfort were the cause of her falls. At that point, the care team agreed to keep her pain medications to a minimum.

Grace began to decline. She moved less, she "spoke" less. There were subtle changes in her behavior. Her physical evaluation (labs, exam) turned up normal. Yet Grace was losing weight. Another care plan was developed, and her case was discussed at the next Weight Loss Committee meeting. She was placed on supplements. She was placed on an appetite stimulant.

Given the high blood pressure that is associated with diabetes, she took medications to help control her blood sugars. She wanted to eat, but she did not want to eat the food that was given to her. She began to steal sweets and snacks from the rooms of other residents. Two new care plans were developed, the first to manage her diabetes and the second to manage her behavior.

Under the first new care plan, her blood sugar medications were adjusted, and her diet was more strictly controlled. (She still did not eat everything on her diabetic food trays, but her blood sugars did lower.)

To deal with Grace's habit of stealing food, a psychiatrist saw her and placed her on an anticompulsive medication. Other residents were advised to hide their treats. The eating of unauthorized food stopped.

Grace continued to lose weight. Despite many interventions, including an appetite stimulant, she continued to decline. Her dementia had advanced to such a degree that she had forgotten how to eat and required help. Artificially fed, her body was still failing. More and more, she was bed-bound. She developed pressure areas on her heel. Skin breakdown is "flagged" as a serious problem in the long-term care facility. It is penalized in surveys. Another care plan was developed. Special mattresses and a turning schedule were developed. She was given extra vitamins. However, she continued to do poorly and experience more breakdowns in her skin. I was asked to write a statement of "unavoidability," which I did, as such deterioration is indeed part of the dying process and truly unavoidable.

Grace's daughters remained attentive and involved in her care. However, they were not realistic about her prognosis. Grace could not be cured. She could be made comfortable, fed, and bathed. It was possible, too, to control her blood pressure and to treat her diabetes with pills. Only her mind would never return. Still, Mrs. Comas-Diaz's daughters remained determined to "cure" their mother. Many times I conversed with them regarding their mother's prognosis and treatment options, which remained limited. They did not seem to understand that Mom, at best, would remain the same, and most likely decline. The staff reinforced my opinion and spoke to the women about the natural process of end-stage dementia, to no avail. Grace's daughters perceived care as curing; easing symptoms was beside the point.

Grace, meanwhile, had several episodes of pneumonia, each of the sort that could easily be treated in the nursing home with outcomes as good, if not better, than at a hospital. Her daughters did not agree. With each bout of pneumonia, they insisted that Grace go to the hospital. When she was no longer able to swallow food very well (although she was able to eat soft things), her children arranged for the installation of a feeding tube. Her younger daughter, however, continued to coax her to eat without the tube—to make her normal again. One day Grace choked on her food and needed to be re-hospitalized.

Grace became weaker and more confused after each trip out of the facility. Her girls did not seem able to make the connection between transferring this frail woman, with no hope for a cure and an altered perception of peoples' actions (due to her dementia), and the continued decline in her mental and physical status.

As far as I could tell, intravenous lines and blood draws were torture to Grace. A new environment left her more insecure and disoriented than ever. She had little reserve for change. I explained this to her daughters, as did the nursing staff and administration. We made no impression.

The family continued to want aggressive treatment and a "cure" for Grace. Diligent documentation of aggressive care appeared in Grace's chart. Her daughters insisted on weekly laboratory studies. Although neither woman had a medical background, each demanded copies of all of their mother's blood work when they called me for an update.

Grace developed an infection. Her daughters sent her to the hospital. She developed another infection, and they sent her to the hospital again. The cycle continued for more than a year and involved nine hospitalizations.

Despite adequate care plans and management, Grace was dying. She was unresponsive and did not recognize anyone. Devoid of human expression, she did not smile. A care plan for her death was developed. Grace was not allowed to die without one.

To the end, the family continued to insist on aggressive measures. To treat every infection or fever that Grace experienced, she was sent per family instructions to the emergency room. She was headed there one night when, at long last, she died in the ambulance. She was among strangers. Her daughters had driven on ahead to meet her at the hospital.

Grace's management is an example of what I call a care plan "tree" or a "cascade" of care plans: One care plan leads to another. Solving one problem only leads to more difficulties—as well as care plans.

What was the outcome for Grace? Were pain, falls, weight loss, skin breakdown, sepsis, and her death preventable? Was Grace comfortable? Were we too involved in the care plans to look at their futility? Who was happy? Grace showed no emotions. Neither happiness, nor its opposite, was something she could express. Certainly her family was not happy—Grace was not cured. The care team was not happy—we were too busy writing care plans.

Grace—The Social Model

From the standpoint of the Social Management System, Grace was a desirable resident.

She had a terminal diagnosis. Actually, she had several of them, including end-stage dementia and vascular disease. Treatment options were also very limited and of questionable benefit. Ironically, she also suffered from several inadvertent problems, which caused both morbidity and mortality, as the result of the diagnostic process and the "attempted" treatment processes.

What Grace really needed was increased support from caregivers in the form of creature comforts and the solace of human presence. Hospice could have effectively treated Grace's discomfort at the end of life and perhaps allowed her to feel more at ease with the dying process. Despite advanced dementia, she could have benefited from human companionship; the human touch. Instead she was in pain and distress. Palliative medications could have been administered, but her daughters refused to authorize any, fearing over-sedation.

Though unacknowledged, Grace's family needed support during the dying process as well. Her children had lost their father shortly before Grace's admittance into long-term care. Now they hid from their own anguish in a relentless pursuit of medical appointments for their mother. Natural grieving never occurred. Although hospice could have provided the daughters with counseling and spiritual support, they denied that their mother lay dying, and argued instead that her decline was the result of poor care.

Hospice could have provided Grace with equipment to add to her comfort at the end of her life, such as a special bed and wheelchair that her family could not afford. Her daughters opted instead for treatments with expensive antibiotics and intravenous fluids (both of which were covered by insurance).

Grace's situation was just the sort that the Social Management System was designed to address. Yet her family did not accept this model. All attempts to persuade them otherwise were futile. Instead, Grace received less than optimal care, per family request. Long-term care is a business and, of course, "the customer is always right." Indeed only the family's wishes were served by the ill-chosen scientific model in Grace's case. Even so, her daughters missed out on the support that hospice would have provided, freeing them to spend much more time with their mother.

The staff, of course, could have given Grace more care, had they not been required to spend so much time administering so many care plans. The facility administrators would have been better off as well. Care would have been less costly, and the outcome better in terms of the level of risk of legal liability. All would have benefited, except the family, who simply would not accept that medical science could not save their mother.

Grace—The Business Model

Grace was an undesirable resident from the standpoint of the Business Management System. She had insurance when she was admitted, lost her insurance, was private pay, and had multiple payers after each hospitalization. Although eventually reimbursed, the facility did not have a consistent source of payment, and changes in her insurance plans often delayed payments. From a financial standpoint, Grace's care required a significant amount of time on the part of the billing office (which had to hire a specialized worker paid by the hour) to get proper payment.

She was in the hospital so often that her room was unoccupied for a significant period of time. Although the facility was not receiving steady payment from Grace's insurance, the administrators could not market her bed to anyone else, as she was still a resident and not officially discharged. While she was in the hospital, she "held" her bed, which she was allowed to do by law for a certain number of days.

Her advanced age was another disadvantage from a business standpoint. Under the best of circumstances, Mrs. Comas-Diaz would only live in the facility a short time (statistically), given her age. A new resident would have to be found to take her place. Her room would be empty for at least a short time, and revenues would be lost. Meanwhile, she underwent many expensive treatments. She had a feeding tube and received intravenous antibiotics and fluids at multiple points in time. For the facility, these treatments incurred added expenses in terms of labor (nursing staff) as well as an expensive pharmacy bill, not totally covered by her insurance.

Grace also was a very high risk from a legal standpoint. Dissatisfied with her status, her family threatened to sue the facility early on. State surveyors were not pleased about her problems (wounds, diabetes, infections, weight loss), nor with the multiple care plans meant to deal with them. Proper documentation was a constant concern. Nor did Mrs. Comas-Diaz have "connections" to other facilities or to a retirement community to provide referral sources. She was an isolated resident, referred by her own family. She would not bring further business to the facility.

If the business model benefited neither Grace nor the facility, it did benefit Grace's family. Ironically, her insurance covered expensive intravenous therapies but refused to pay for a comfortable bed that would have relieved the pain of her bedsores. She was on Medicare by the time she began receiving expensive antibiotics, tube feedings, and diagnostic testing. After her Medicare was exhausted, she used Medicaid for her long-term care stay. The cycle would continue with each hospitalization.

Grace—The Ethical Model

Grace was unable to give consent or to ask for treatment. However, her plan of acute care should have provided her family with a consistent source of information on a regular basis. Instead, Grace's family received most information about her case during crisis situations. They would talk to the emergency room doctor, whom they would see only once. Grace would be taken care of by new physicians and nurses each time she was admitted to the hospital. The family would ask their opinions. Of course, none of these professionals knew what Grace's life was really like. Many perhaps did not even know that she resided at a long-term care facility. They relied on information from her family alone. Once each crisis passed, the family waited until the next problem arose.

Under the ethical model, information is offered to residents and their families on a consistent basis to enable them to make informed decisions about health care. In the case of Graciella Comas-Diaz, the care team fulfilled this obligation and informed her family of the futility of further medical treatment. In principle, Grace had the right to refuse treatment and to seek human comfort at the end of her life. In fact, however, once her daughters made an informed decision to deny their mother's terminal condition, it became the ethical duty of the care team to carry out their wishes.

10

Insurance and the Absurd

We create systems to benefit the elderly and the chronically ill, yet the systems develop a life of their own. They dictate courses of action that sometimes are contrary to our original ideas. We put faith in these systems to such an extent that we no longer question the outcomes. The dental woes of two very different residents illustrate the point.

Rock 'n Roll Dentures

After a life of travel in a heavy metal band, Frank Olympia came to live at Fern Oakes when he was about forty-five. He suffered from multiple sclerosis and had attempted suicide. At the facility, he made some psychological and emotional adjustments, which improved his quality of life, and he remained mentally alert.

Frank was in need of dental care. Some teeth needed to be filled, while others needed to come out. His dental insurance would pay for complete extractions and dentures but not for restorative dental work, such as fillings and crowns. Not yet fifty, Frank was unhappy at the prospect of losing all of his teeth. He decided to seek a second opinion and scheduled an appointment with another dentist. In the meantime, he began to experience immense dental pain. I offered to prescribe a medication, but Frank was reluctant to take it. He had a long history of narcotic abuse and dependence, which he had worked hard to overcome and did not want to jeopardize.

In the end, the pain became too much. Frank took the medication that I prescribed and managed not to abuse it. He went in for the second opinion about his teeth on a hopeful note, willing to pay for restorative dental work out of pocket. Unfortunately, the cost was well beyond him. Restoration of his teeth would cost him upward of eight thousand dollars. Reluctantly, he underwent the complete extractions and obtained dentures; his insurance paid in full.

Bad Bite, Too Bad

As you may recall, Katie Collins entered long-term care when she was about eighty-five, having functioned well in an assisted-living setting for the previous five years. Part of the gradual decline in Katie's functional status resulted from her weight loss. The facility care team approached me to ask: Does she need a feeding tube or an appetite stimulant? Should we send her to a specialist for a work-up? Perhaps she has a hidden cancer?

I ordered some basic labs and diagnostic testing. The results came back normal.

A few weeks later, the nursing supervisor approached me.

"Katie's still losing weight," she said. "You've got to put something in her chart—to document the unavoidability of her weight loss."

"What do you mean?" I asked.

"I mean she'll raise a red flag," the supervisor said.

The state and city inspectors were due into the facility any day.

I called Mrs. Collins's daughter. Quite irate, she filled me in on the details, which the care team had failed to tell me. Because her dentures no longer fit, Katie had begun to eat without them. The new soft food diet was not high enough in calories, however, to permit her to maintain her weight. New dentures seemed to be the solution. The difficulty was that her insurance paid for new ones only once every five years. Unfortunately, she had purchased the ill-fitting pair more recently than that. A new set would cost her more than five thousand dollars, which her family could not afford. As the problem was not resolved, Katie continued to lose weight.

Apparently, the care team had bullied her daughter a bit. "Either Mom starts eating more, or they say they're going to put in a feeding tube or send her to hospice," she told me.

Insurance would cover feeding tube placement, as well as artificial feedings (which, incidentally, would be much more expensive than dentures).

"Is there some way you could talk to the insurance company about getting new dentures?" Katie's daughter asked me.

It took some time, but the insurance company did come round to recognize the special circumstances. The company did agree to pay half the cost, and the family picked up the remainder.

Katie got her teeth. She began to eat. Everyone was happy.

In the cases of Frank and Katie, the common ingredient was more than the need for dental care. Each depended on a less obvious common denominator, namely, the business system, ostensibly created to help people cope with the unexpected. Yet the purveyors of such insurance apply their own broad rules without necessary regard for the outcome in the individual case. In what appears to have been a random reconsideration of the rules, Frank lost out, whereas Katie won an exemption.

No doubt, Frank had no one to blame but himself for poor dental hygiene, yet the absurdity of applying an insurance model developed for an elder at the end of life to a relatively young adult is obvious. (Frank's insurance would not pay to clean his teeth, but it would pay to pull them out and replace them with dentures.)

On the other hand, Katie's need for dentures was not the result of some fault of her own. Dentures are common among today's elders, who lived a good part of their lives before the fluoridation of water. If ever there was a case where modern-era insurance should be perfectly useful, this need for dentures among the elderly would seem to be it. Yet despite the efforts of many bright people, the insurance industry remains ridiculously inflexible when faced with novel circumstances. Until I intervened, Katie's insurance company had been predisposed to pay for the installation of a far more expensive and intrusive feeding tube to help her maintain her weight rather than revoke its "five-year plan" and pay for a new set of dentures. Eventually at least, the company did agree that the new dentures would accomplish the same goal much more easily and cheaply and, need we say, in a more natural fashion.

Vanity in Vain

Rose Jamison, as you will recall, came to the facility when she was eighty-two and in an advanced stage of Parkinson's disease. A proud woman, part of Mrs. Jamison's problems with home care was her unwillingness to use such aids as a walker, a special toilet seat, or large padded spoons to help in her feeding.

Mrs. Jamison was also quite vain. She could not hear well but refused to try a hearing aid. Although she did undergo surgery to remove cataracts, she missed out on movies and did not read because she was unwilling to wear eyeglasses.

Mrs. Jamison had chronic headaches. Nothing seemed to help. She came to the conclusion that sinus troubles were the symptom and that her oddly shaped nose and her overbite were the cause. It was always possible that her self-diagnosis was accurate. Yet, here she was, an elderly woman who had never experienced such problems before. Still, Mrs. Jamison was certain: Rhinoplasty (a nose job) and orthodonture (braces) would cure her. She did some "shopping" and found a doctor that would do the surgery and document the justification properly so that insurance would pay. She also got braces. In the end, Mrs. Jamison's nose was a bit more in fashion, and her teeth were straight. Her headaches, however, remained.

Later on, Mrs. Jamison developed back pain. I treated her with physical therapy, analgesics, and anti-inflammatory drugs. The regimen only made her feel worse, she told me. She went on to see a chiropractor and an acupuncture specialist, who could not help her. From there, she proceeded to a neurologist, a physiatrist, and an orthopedic surgeon, all of whom ordered multiple tests. None produced a diagnosis.

It was only as Rose was preparing to go to the Senior Ball that she hit on the cause of her back pain. While trying on various gowns, she got several good looks at her undressed body in the mirror. It was then that it dawned on her. Her breasts! Sagging and pendulous, they were the problem. Her poor, frail back could not support them. Breast-reduction surgery and implants were medically indicated, and there was a surgeon to be found who would agree. At the Senior Ball, Rose was crowned "prom queen," but her back pain did not disappear.

Despite her attractive teeth, nose, and breasts, Mrs. Jamison died a few years later. Her death was unrelated to her sinus problems, headaches, or back pain. She was old, and her body had worn itself out in the long struggle with Parkinson's disease.

As a postscript, I met Mrs. Jamison's daughter Emma at a local salon some months after her mother's death. I was there to buy shampoo. Emma was there to pay for a "makeover" that her teenaged daughter had just had in preparation for the school dance that evening. Standing in line behind the two of them, I could not help but overhear the receptionist charge Emma two hundred and fifty dollars, an expenditure in keeping with Rose's own penchants, although a bit profligate for my tastes. Still it was not my concern. The three of us parted cordially, and I gave the matter not another thought.

A week or so later, my billing company called me. The Jamison family owed me fifteen dollars, which insurance had not covered, for my last visit to see Rose before she passed. If my recollection was right, I had scheduled a special meeting with the family to discuss their questions and concerns. I had spent well over thirty-five minutes with them, and I had answered many phone calls during Mrs. Jamison's final days. Now my billing representative was telling me that Mrs. Jamison's eldest daughter, Julie, had telephoned to say that the family would not pay the bill, because "Mom was dead." Did I want to send the bill on to collections or write it off?

Believe in Braces
Although the nursing home is notorious, we can find ample examples in our modern lives, where scientific, social, and business models lure us into arrangements that seem based in progress and reason, yet, on more careful scrutiny, prove to constitute a rigid and unquestioned structure. Although the trappings may look and feel good, the overarching system and its structure are actually mechanical, uncaring, and shallow. Such a description may apply to our workplace, our local schools, condominium board, and not just to the LTC facility.

Which brings me to braces. I began to go to the dentist in the mid-sixties, when fluorinated toothpaste, dental floss, and sealants came into use widely. Mine was the first generation that could be cavity free, or close to it, through diligent self-care with these modern products and a biannual trip to the dentist for professional cleaning. Orthodonture also began to become popular. I was not even considered a candidate for this procedure, as my teeth, although not perfect, were close enough. Given the few orthodontists at the time, their job was to take care of those who truly needed help.

Thirty years later, orthodonture is covered by insurance offered to many employees. The number of orthodontists has grown by leaps and bounds. All of a sudden, our kids are almost "required" to have teeth that look like those that belong to movie stars and models. It is not uncommon these days for a child to be referred to an orthodontist for a very slight "imperfection" (or, as some would argue—an individual look) at a very, very young age. In fact, I have seen statistics that ninety-five percent of children need orthodontics, and thus parents are urged to obtain the necessary insurance.

What do "necessary" and "need" mean in this case? Less than perfect teeth are rarely a threat to health. Yet many people choose to straighten their teeth by wearing braces in their twenties, thirties, forties, and sometimes even much later. I know someone who had braces put on at the age of fifty-nine, not to mention Rose Jamison who did the same at eighty-plus. (Of course the elderly Rose's several cosmetic surgeries fairly beg the question of how we define need.)

What really should be said is that people in the business of dentistry and affiliated fields, such as dental education, tacitly recognize that braces are beneficial to their systems. Businesses sell more insurance to cover the cost with little risk. (Rarely is anyone harmed by wearing braces—and rarely is anyone sued for providing them.)

Dental schools train highly educated and skilled persons whom the society at large later employs as highly paid professionals. As part of the related social system, we are expected to accept the notion that cosmetic dental care likewise benefits us. If, through insurance coverage, we are offered a benefit (say, braces) and the cost to obtain it is relatively insignificant, we are expected to accept it. What was once an optional luxury and a personal choice almost becomes a requirement. Once the beliefs in a need and a benefit are in place, they become hard to resist. Even if one has the strength and conviction to be a part of a small minority, the nagging questions linger: Why do all these other people choose to change their appearance in this way? Am I a bad mother for not offering the "best" to my child?

Not surprisingly, putting braces on a child's teeth has become a popular way for a parent to show that she cares. The parent is happy, as she has given her child a chance to look "her best." Little effort or time needs to be put into this demonstration of affection, if insurance covers the charges, and all Mom has to do is to chauffeur—or ask the babysitter or nanny to drive—back and forth to the appointments. The school system, meanwhile, allows children to leave school routinely to go to the orthodontist but does not excuse them to take the afternoon off to visit with out-of-town grandparents.

Sometimes, however, the optional nature of what we have come to see as an absolute need resurfaces. Even in the case of orthodonture such a glimpse at reality can occur.

Take, for instance, my daughter's friend Sarah, who has poor dentition and wants braces. Sarah is the only child of divorced parents. Her mother is a successful, self-employed advertising agent, who pays for health insurance but not for dental insurance because it is too expensive. A biannual trip by her daughter to the dentist costs more than two hundred dollars. Sarah's mom is quite willing to pay this amount for her daughter's routine cleanings. To pay thousands of dollars for braces is another matter. It would come down to a choice: braces or a good education. Public school in their neighborhood is sub-par, and Sarah's mother pays private school tuition. Straightening Sarah's teeth can wait.

Even after biannual cleanings and fluoridated water, our kids still get cavities and need fillings. Why? Well, it takes both time and effort to ensure that your child actually does a thorough job of brushing. It takes emotional energy to withstand with good humor and composure their crying fits when they insist on candy. Oral hygiene and a healthy diet take personal responsibility. They do not, however, benefit the medical, business, or social models. In fact, we will use those models less if we rely on ourselves more.

Do we see certain discrepancies here?

We have surrendered our personal responsibilities to the systems that run business, medicine, and popular culture. Do we believe in these systems so fervently that we do not have to admit that we have given up our autonomy to them?

In summary: "Need" is reached by a consensus based on scientific knowledge, public beliefs and expectations, and available finances. "Caring" is defined based on prevailing social norms, science, and the payer source. "Options" are limited by what is paid for, which, in turn, is determined by the definition of the "need" above and not necessarily by what we really require. What is paid for, in accordance with the doctrine of the management system, might be the more expensive and less intuitive option.

11

Loneliness and the Mail Order Catalog

I travel to my third facility, Grove Court, about ten minutes away in time from Sweet Penny Tree, but a million miles away in mindset. I go there once a month to see a few residents. The facility is in an upscale part of town and reflects that socioeconomic fact. Many of the residents are retired doctors, lawyers, and businessmen. Some are women with alcoholic dementia, married to—or divorced from—such men.

On the way there, I receive several calls. The first is from a funeral director. He needs me to sign a death certificate for direct cremation. We arrange for a place to meet.

The next is from a nurse at Sonoma Ranch. "Jody Miller's son died unexpectedly," the nurse tells me of one of my elderly patients. "Her daughter is coming in this morning to give her the news. Could you prescribe a sedative in case she needs one?"

Of course I can, although I want to cry. Jody dotes on her children.

The last call is a kind that I dread. It is from the administrator at the Wentworth facility. "Our census is low," she says, meaning that there are empty beds. "Do you have a patient or two that you can send us?"

"I'll think about it," I say, although I do not enjoy the idea of hustling little old ladies, nor do I wish to lure people into institutional living as long as they can possibly avoid it. I pull into the parking lot, guarded by a couple of stone lions. Grove Court is top-notch, at least when it comes to décor.

Never treated very well by the staff, I am treated no better this morning. I walk in, and the two aides leaning against the receptionist's station act like they have never seen me before, although of course they have. One of them is a real joker, who often goes out of his way to aggravate me, walking off with my patients' charts or misplacing them when he knows that I need them. I nod and say good morning to them in any case.

Most Grove Court residents are quite formal and respond cautiously to behavior that might be considered casual, let alone spontaneous. A few really do want me as their doctor. That is why I continue to come here.

The four residents whom I will see today, however, are not quite capable of giving me a warm welcome. The first is Doris, a woman with end-stage dementia. Recently, she was put on a feeding tube, and her family decided to designate her care as hospice. She is nonverbal and bed-bound.

The second resident has advanced dementia. She walks and talks but has no idea what she is saying or where she is going. She has the same unusual name as I do. Each time I see her, I say, "Hello, Gilah."

"Hello," she returns my greeting. She sounds unsure of herself.

"Do you know my name?"

She shakes her head no.

"It's Gilah. Just you like yours!"

Gilah's face lights up, as though she is beginning to understand something wonderful. "Dr. Gilah!" she says and then she laughs.

Each month when I come to visit her (now going on five years), we reenact this scene together. No matter how much I dread Groves Court, I feel good again, once Gilah starts to laugh.

My third resident, Alberto, is sad and slight. His severe vascular disease led to the amputation of both legs a year ago. He tends to weep when I visit him. Always he asks, "When will I be going home?"

Never, from what I understand. His wife has made it clear to us that she does not want him living in the house. I do not believe it would be right for me to relay this information to him. There is some other information, however, that I do need to give him today.

"The second chest x-ray came back abnormal," I tell him. "There's a strong chance that you have lung cancer."

Alberto does not seem to care.

Out at the nurses' station, I drop off his x-ray.

"Could you order a psych evaluation for him?" the nurse asks me. "He cries to go home so much of the time."

What I take as a show of concern encourages me. "Has anyone told Alberto that his wife will not take him back home?"

"I don't know what you mean," she replies.

"His wife won't take him back," I repeat.

She gives me a blank stare.

And now there is my fourth resident, Marion. A rich lady with no family, her only relative was a sister who passed away several years ago. At ninety-three, she came to Grove Court after she fell and hit her head and required surgery. That was two years ago.

Marion was quite difficult to get to know. She hears nearly nothing. Every time I pay her a visit, we go through the same scenario, one that is far less fun than the one I go through with Gilah. When I enter her room, Marion never has her hearing device (called a pocket talker), and we spend a few minutes locating it. Invariably, the device has no batteries.

"Look through my dresser." She raises her voice to a high, loud pitch and must assume that I cannot hear any better than she can. I find no batteries. I should be patient, but I am annoyed.

"Use my writing board," she bellows. Her pen has no ink.

"Why do you want to speak to me," she continues to yell. "I can't hear you, anyway, and I don't know who you are."

She does know who I am. Marion is quite lucid, if excitable.

After rifling through her dresser again, I do find a battery, and I pull a pen out of my own bag. Finally, the pocket talker and the writing board are working. Marion calms down. So do I.

I ask how she is doing.

"I need a prescription filled," she says. "Wait a minute, and I'll show you." Once again, the dresser drawers are ransacked until she finds what she is looking for, an advertisement from a magazine about an arthritic cream. It is an over-the-counter medication.

"You don't need a prescription," I tell her. "Mr. Walsh can buy it at the drugstore and bring it in to you."

The mention of her guardian's name brings on a sigh. "Why can't I go home?" she asks.

"It's not up to me. It's up to Mr. Walsh," I tell her, just as I have many times.

"Well, it's awfully depressing," she tells me. "I'm not like the others, you know. They've lost their minds, or else their arms or their legs. I do feel very sorry for them, but it's not my cup of tea to keep them company."

She worries about how she will get her taxes done.

"You have a lawyer and a guardian to take care of them," I remind her.

She needs to get her late sister Dottie's personal belongings in order.

"I want to move down to Florida. Not this year. I missed this year. But next time. I can live down there on my own and sort out her affairs."

I listen without comment. In a moment she changes the subject.

"I don't like the air conditioning in here—do you? It's cold. I can't live in air conditioning."

Suddenly she is talking about her childhood. "Papa always wanted me to be a boy. I tried to please him. He was a picky eater—have I told you that? Well, he was. I only ate what he ate. To please him. That's why I'm a picky eater now."

She is offering me a clue, perhaps. She has been losing weight steadily for some time.

"Mother died at an early age, and father married a younger woman. One night I came home late to dinner. That woman boxed my ears!" She jabs a finger at each ear. "She beat the sound right out. After that—well, after that—Dottie always made fun of me."

It is time for me to say good-bye. Marion does not want me to leave. I squeeze her hand.

As I exit, the staff has returned to the floor. I hand Marion's chart to a nurse's aide, who rolls her eyes and smirks when she sees the name. "That woman is something else," she says. "Her joy in life is buying things out of catalogs. Last month, she bought herself a wig and a bikini—can you believe it?" The aide chuckles at her recollection. "Her guardian is putting a stop to it, thank God."

I can only nod without enthusiasm. What she says makes me sad.

I leave the building. As I cross the parking lot, I hear someone's heels clicking on the pavement behind me. I turn to see the nurse's aide, running to catch up to me. In her arms is a clutch of catalogs.

"Hold on there, doctor," she calls. "I want to show you something." As she reaches me, she slaps the catalogs down on the hood of my car, where they fan out rather decoratively.

"See what I mean," she says. "They're all addressed to Marion."

I glance down. So they are.

"I just wanted you to know that I've been saving your patient lots of money," she says with pride. "When the mail comes in, I go through and weed out most of the catalogs, see, especially the ones with the expensive merchandise. That way, she only gets one or two of them a month. It's like damage control," She gives me a grin. "She gets tons of these things," the aide goes on, as if she were not sure that I understood the good deed she was performing.

She is quite right. I do not understand. I feel only pity to learn that lonely Marion's last remaining pleasures in life is being curtailed. I think, too, of the evening pleasure that I will have, browsing an online catalog for bargains. I may not even buy anything. Just looking keeps me going.

12

All in the Family

In ideal circumstances, families look after their own. Even when they do not, they wield considerable influence over how residents fare. Typically, the family falls into one of the same categories as the care team does.

- The normal family
- The bickering (dysfunctional) family
- The absent family
- The passive (holiday) family
- No family
- The threatening family

Like a care team, one family alone can move through all six categories as circumstances and stress levels change over time. Charles Smith's family provides an example.

Charles Smith arrived at Sweet Penny Tree one afternoon not the least bit aware that he had just arrived at his new home. That morning, one of his three sons had packed a suitcase for his dad and helped him into the car.

"I told him we were coming here to see Mom," his youngest son, Jack, told me later.

Mr. Smith's wife, Vera, was a short-term resident at Sweet Penny Tree, undergoing rehabilitation for a fractured hip after a fall. Several weeks into her three-month stay, her husband was happy to visit her there. At eighty-seven, Charles Smith had advancing Parkinson's disease, mild dementia, and a history of seizures. He had leaned heavily on his wife for care, which included daily administration of a dozen medications. Once she fell, however, new arrangements were needed.

Vera understood that her husband was entering Sweet Penny Tree as a resident. Only Charles himself was left in the dark. Perhaps his family feared that he would be upset and not understand. For whatever reason, his wife and her sons chose not to tell Charles that he was now a permanent resident.

Saturday morning dawned, and Mr. Smith awoke in the facility, alone and confused. He had trouble eating his breakfast and choked on his food. He also had trouble walking, which did not deter him from wandering. Throughout the morning, different staff members found him weaving his way uncertainly along the corridors of the facility. Each time, they led Mr. Smith back to his room. Each time, he went out again to roam.

"I'm going home," he told everyone he met. In his search for an exit, he entered the women's bathing area, which created an uproar.

By the time that I arrived in mid-afternoon, several staff members, as well as the director of nursing, were waiting to see me. I was given a list of concerns to evaluate and address before I had even seen Mr. Smith. Should he be sent to the emergency room? Should a nurse call the psychiatrist? Or should I order sedatives for him? Opinions varied.

In his room I found Mr. Smith resting. He looked tired after his morning trek through the halls. The chair in which he sat was a special one with an alarm that would go off if he were to get up again on his own. I reviewed his chart and old records. The results of tests that I had ordered earlier that day were largely normal. For his part, Mr. Smith appeared comfortable and voiced no complaints. His eyes held for me a question but no anger. I had little else to go on, as his mental state meant that I could perform only a limited exam—he had trouble understanding and cooperating with me. From what I did see, though, there were no physical abnormalities.

In all probability, Mr. Smith was experiencing delirium as a result of the change in his environment. I would allow him time to adjust to the facility. Perhaps his delirium would clear on its own. If not, I would make some adjustments in his regimen. I discussed my plan with the nurses. The situation was not unusual. We had dealt with similar cases many times.

How would a normal, (that is, a healthy) family help Mr. Smith?

The normal family acts as a patient advocate. Family members are receptive to information that they receive from the physician, nurses, social workers, and other staff. They take such information into account and use it to make decisions on behalf of the resident family member. They also take into account the resident's personal choices and act upon them.

As I was leaving the facility, Mr. Smith's family arrived. They had come not to see Mr. Smith but to pick up his wife. Vera was well enough to attend her granddaughter's bridal shower, which was about to begin in an hour.

"We'd like to talk to you about Dad when it's convenient," Jack said.

Though it was Saturday afternoon, I offered to meet with the family there and then. The wedding that weekend offered a rare opportunity to meet the extended family, if for a short time. In addition to Vera, Jack, and his wife, I could speak directly with Terry, the eldest of Mr. Smith's three sons, who lived in New York.

"Poor Chuck," Vera said. "He's more confused than ever."

Confusion and regression are not uncommon when an elderly, ill person moves into a new environment. Physical and mental reserves are small.

"His medications may be contributing to his confusion," I said to Vera. "Only I don't want to change anything at this point. It might only add to his confusion. This is an adjustment period; let's wait and see how he does."

Jack filled me in on some medical history of his dad's that was not in the records. What he said was helpful and informative. Though there was nothing life-threatening or critical to worry about at the moment, I did ask about Charles' wishes regarding health care. Would he want measures taken such as mechanical ventilation and insertion of a feeding tube?

"Definitely not," Jack said. "My father would not want any of those things."

"You'll need to sign some papers then," I told him. Jack was the son who had power of attorney over his father's affairs.

"My brother Tom will probably want to talk to you too," Jack said. "He lives in Colorado and couldn't make it to the wedding."

I gave Jack my telephone number. "Have Tom call me any time."

We parted after about a twenty-minute conversation. Everyone seemed satisfied with the situation. The Smiths agreed to wait a few weeks to see how Charles adjusted to the new environment. After he became acclimatized, I would send him to a neurologist. In the meantime, I discussed strategies to help Mr. Smith adjust to the "lifestyle" change.

To make him feel more at home, Jack brought in family photos and a few of his dad's golf trophies. Despite his initial lack of communication with his father about his placement at Sweet Penny Tree, Jack was proving to be quite supportive. He visited on a daily basis.

Vera, meanwhile, completed her rehab successfully and returned home, clearly relieved to be spared the day-to-day care of her husband, which had been taxing for some time. Now she visited Chuck every day at Sweet Penny Tree, where the two had dinner together and watched movies. Gradually, Mr. Smith returned to his baseline. Though Parkinson's continued to impair him, he was able to enjoy television, meal times, and the company of his wife and his local son. The Smiths were content, as was the care team, which had been as cooperative and attentive as the Smiths themselves. Mr. Smith smiled!

In the weeks that followed, however, time and distance began to take their toll. For logistical reasons, the eldest son, Terry, had relinquished legal responsibility for his father's affairs to his youngest brother, Jack. Yet Terry was not happy to have done so. He lacked confidence in Jack, and he found the distance between him and the facility a constant source of frustration. Before long, the brothers no longer agreed on treatment for their dad. Their disagreements began to affect their father's care.

How would a bickering, that is, a dysfunctional, family affect Mr. Smith?

The bickering (dysfunctional) family is in conflict on proper care. No one person serves as a point of contact, available to receive information from the facility and to disseminate it to other family members in a consistent manner. In the absence of consensus, information received from the staff is circulated among the family members in a disjointed way and often misinterpreted. Family members often trade contradictory or conflicting information concerning care.

ॐ

One afternoon I received a call from Terry. "I'm concerned about the nursing care my father is getting," he said.

"What do you see as the problem?" I asked.

"I don't like the attitude when I call. The nurse I talked to last night acted like my father was a moron."

"Well, that's not good," I agreed. "I'll speak to the director of nursing."

A few hours later, Jack called

"How's Dad doing, Doctor? I've been traveling and couldn't make it in to see him."

"Your dad's doing fine," I said. "I heard from your brother Terry earlier this evening."

"Oh, really?" Jack seemed surprised.

"Terry's concerned about your dad's nursing care."

"How can he tell? He's not here to see what's going on. I think the nursing care is fine."

"From what I understand, it's an attitude problem he's encountering at the nursing station."

"Attitude problem. He's the one with one of those." I could hear Jack snort.

"Your dad's stable," I replied. "I won't need to see him again until Monday."

"That's good to hear," Jack said. "And, say, I wouldn't take Terry too seriously. He's always been touchy."

On Saturday morning Terry called me again. He was quite irate.

"Jack told me Dad needs minimal medical care."

"I wouldn't say that, but it's true that your father is doing fine."

"I question that, Doctor. Dad is in terrible shape. You've got to do something."

"I'm puzzled to hear you say that. Your mother seems to think he's returned to his old self."

"He's totally out of it. I don't think he even knows who I am when I call."

"Your mother tells me he's been confused for some time. He doesn't recognize her voice on the phone, either."

"See, he's going downhill. I'd like him tested further."

"We can do further tests," I said, although the testing done thus far had revealed no particular problem. As we continued our conversation, it became clear that, until the weekend of the wedding, Terry had not seen his father in more than seven years.

On Monday, Jack arrived just as I finished examining his dad.

"How's he doing?"

"He's about the same. Terry would like to do further neurological tests."

"He would? Well, what does he know?"

"In any case, I think that we should wait a bit longer. As I've mentioned, confusion and regression are not uncommon in a new environment. As you both know, I did order some lab tests to rule out an acute illness as a cause of your father's problems."

Jack nodded. "I'll sign those papers not to resuscitate Dad while I'm here." They had been waiting for his signature.

"Have you discussed the DNR with Terry?" I asked. "He didn't want it signed when I last spoke to him."

Jack's face grew red. "Why the hell not? I'm sick and tired of all the responsibility. Tom is missing in action, and Terry undercuts everything I do. I'm fed up."

It was true that I had heard nothing from or about Tom. As for Jack and Terry, I noticed that they did not seem to communicate with each other very much. They tended to leave their conflicts for others to sort out. In the Smiths' case, much of the family strife arose from the absence from the scene of two out of three children.

How would the absence of family members affect Mr. Smith?
The absent family is generally unavailable to the patient and to the health care team. Care is difficult to give because decisions and consent are difficult to obtain. Developing a care plan is a lengthy,

drawn-out process and, under the circumstances, often does not benefit the resident.

Terry continued to call with a variety of requests, most of which Jack vetoed. Tom did not appear to be in touch with the family at all. Given the geographic distances among the brothers and their differences of opinion about their father's care, I told Jack that a family meeting might be in order. "If your brothers can't travel, we could do a conference call."

With great difficulty, the brothers came up with a time to meet via conference call in the month ahead, which took into account their various constraints and demands. In the interim, the DNR papers were left unsigned, and further tests were put off, too. Vera grew too frail to drive to the facility every day, and Jack begged off more and more.

"I don't have time to see you next week," I heard Jack say to his dad when I came in to check on Mr. Smith. "I won't have time to drive Vera in to visit, either."

When I spoke to him on the phone a week later, Jack admitted to weariness and resentment. "I'm not going to let Terry second-guess my every move. I'm not going to pick up the slack for Tom."

"Your dad loves to see you and Vera," I replied.

"Don't guilt-trip me, Doctor." Jack hung up.

Whatever his reasons, Jack was growing as distant as his brothers.

How would passivity affect Mr. Smith?
The passive family is a hybrid of the absent and the threatening family. Family members are often difficult to reach. Yet when they are not informed about their resident's progress, they become irate and threatening. Often, they visit the family member at holidays only; they do not see the resident for three to four months at a time.

It became clear that Mr. Smith missed his wife and son. "Jack," he would call out. "Vera." He became more and more agitated and disruptive in the communal areas. Eventually, I prescribed a low-dose sedative. One evening, Charles fell and broke his hip. The sedative was a contributing factor.

"I'm calling about my father's fall." It was Tom on the phone, from Colorado. "I wish someone had told me how weak he's become," he said of his dad.

"Your brother Jack tells me you've been difficult to reach," I told him.

"Yeah, well, never mind that. Just let me know how the surgery goes, okay? I can't get back there to see him," he went on. "I'm recovering from surgery myself. Oh, and do me a favor, will you? Take what my brothers want done with a large grain of salt."

The surgery on Mr. Smith's hip led to many complications including blood loss, delirium, and infection. He returned to the facility after about a month but continued to do poorly. Jack and Vera visited sporadically. Curiously, Terry had stopped calling me altogether after Mr. Smith broke his hip. I did not hear from Tom again.

Shortly after Mr. Smith's return to Sweet Penny Tree, I called Jack. The family meeting via conference call was scheduled to take place later that week.

"Oh, that's been postponed," Jack told me.

"I'm sorry to hear that," I said. "Mr. Smith's DNR papers are still not signed," I reminded him.

"Does that really matter, Doctor?"

"Well, it could matter," I answered, a little taken aback by Jack's tone. "By now, it's clear that your dad's dementia is progressive. He won't get any better."

Jack sighed. "I've got a lot on my plate, but I'll get over there somehow."

He never did.

A few weeks later, a nurse called to say that Mr. Smith had choked on his food. "He's having trouble breathing."

The nurse and I each called Jack several times but could not reach him. Reluctantly, I called Vera. I hated to upset her, knowing how very ill she was.

"Jack is on the road," his mother said. "I'm so sick myself. I'd need an ambulance to get to the hospital." She began to cry.

Jack used to be so reliable about returning my calls. He used to be so caring and supportive of his dad. What had happened?

"His wife left him," Vera blurted to me on the phone, "so he's burying himself in work."

Absence from the scene had been a chronic problem because Mr. Smith's sons were geographically dispersed. Now, with the further deterioration of his wife's health and the new distance that local son Jack had put between himself and his father, Mr. Smith had, for all practical purposes, no family at all.

How would a lack of family affect Mr. Smith?
When no family exists or is unavailable to consult, the facility staff are left to act as advocates and decision makers for the resident.

Mr. Smith was in severe distress. I had no choice but to send him to the hospital. I telephoned the emergency room staff and asked them to call Jack, too, but they had no luck reaching him, either. Several hours later, Jack did respond to our voice-mail messages. By that time, Mr. Smith had had a feeding tube put in and been admitted to the intensive care unit.

"You could've tried paging me," Jack scolded. "It sounds like you've gone overboard, but I'm in Connecticut. I can't second-guess you, much as I'd like to."

"Without the DNR signature, we had little choice but to do what we did for your father," I said.

This time the course of Mr. Smith's hospitalization was long and complicated. He developed multiple bouts of pneumonia. While undergoing a diagnostic procedure, he had a stroke. Bed-bound, he developed wounds. His wounds caused him pain, and his confinement made him restless. His inability to eat made him anxious. Medications were used to treat his pain and anxiety. After about six weeks, Mr. Smith returned to the facility, still totally dependent on a feeding tube to eat. Unable to walk, he was able to sit upright for only a short time. He smiled at times but did not speak. His quality of life was certainly poor.

Out of the blue, Terry began to call me again. Far from receptive, he let me know that his dissatisfaction with his father's care had only grown since I had last heard from him.

"I've been documenting everything," he said, "and I've consulted an attorney."

How would a threatening family affect Mr. Smith?
The threatening family expresses its frustration by warning that it will take legal or other disciplinary action with respect to the staff or the facility, if it does not get the outcome or care that it wants.

Terry called back to make some demands. "I want you to go over every note with me in my father's chart. I want you to read every single one."

Mr. Smith's chart was thick with notes on physical therapy and social-work-related activities. "Why don't I have the chart faxed to you?" I suggested.

Terry accepted my suggestion. "I'll review the chart, and then I'll want to talk about further tests. They've been put off far too long."

When he called me again, Terry demanded a whole-body MRI and a bone scan.

I explained to him why these tests were not appropriate. "What makes you want your dad to undergo them at this point?"

"Because I believe that you and your staff have been negligent in your care," Terry said. "Dad was never like this before. I won't let him deteriorate without a fight."

He hung up, and I expected him to file a lawsuit.

Not long after we spoke, I received a call from a nurse. The Smith family was requesting a discharge order for Charles to leave Sweet Penny Tree. Apparently, they had decided to switch doctors and facilities.

I called Terry.

"We're all on board now," he said. "I can speak for both my brothers and my mother. I showed Dad's chart to a physician here in Nyack. "He agrees that you, as well as the facility, have been negligent."

"Who is the physician? He's never called me."

"Never mind. Dad's out of your hands now."

Sure enough, Jack showed up at Sweet Penny Tree that very day. Two years after he had first brought his dad to live here, he repacked his father's suitcase and oversaw his departure. Quite feeble, Charles Smith lay on a gurney, still dependent on a feeding tube. As I watched him wheeled out of Sweet Penny Tree, I wondered if Jack had told his father that he was going to a new place to live. He would soon be flown to a new facility in New York near Terry.

Shortly afterward, the administrator at Sweet Penny Tree called Jack. She hoped to learn what the Smith family had found wrong with Mr. Smith's care at her facility.

"No comment," Jack said.

As mentioned earlier, families can be drawn to facilities whose staff members operate in a style that is similar or otherwise compatible with their own. Thus the care team that happens to exist at a facility at a given point in time often will determine what sorts of families place their elderly and ill members there as residents.

On the other hand, families may select a mode of care based not on their ill relative's needs but on what best suits their own convenience or finances. Such was the case with Greg Farmer, a young man who was paralyzed from the neck down after he dove into an empty swimming pool.

Greg entered long-term care at age twenty-nine, after undergoing extensive surgery and five months of rehabilitation. At first his father, who had power of attorney over his son's finances, opted for skilled rehabilitative care and intensive therapy. Greg benefited from this care. After a few months, however, his insurance would continue to pay for only part of his therapy. To avoid having to pay the difference, Greg's dad opted for a less intensive program at a reduced rate. This decision puzzled me, as I knew Greg received compensation for his disability through another insurance policy. The disability checks he received would have amply compensated the family for their outlay for his therapy.

Greg did not do well under the new regimen. He took to his bed. He developed infections and went to the hospital. With each hospitalization, his insurance allowed him more "free" days of therapy. As soon as he felt better, however, the therapy ended, and he withdrew and continued to decline with each setback.

Working Every Angle

One day, his father called me.

"I'm concerned about Greg," he said. "I'd like to see some of his medications cut and then maybe he'd get some of his old energy back."

"You know that Greg benefits tremendously from the additional therapy," I reminded him. "You should consider increasing it again, if you want to see him regain his energy."

Greg's dad was not interested.

As I was not averse to simplifying his son's medications, I gradually stopped many of them over the next few months. Greg did not get worse, but he did not improve either. His pharmacy bill, however, was much reduced. Cutting the costs had been his dad's real motive in calling me, as later became clear.

A few years passed. Greg's assets were exhausted, and he applied for Medicaid. Shortly after he was accepted into the program and had a new payer source, his sister called me.

"Greg was taken off many of the meds he was on—Why is that?"

"I stopped them at your dad's request three years ago," I confirmed.

"Well, Medicaid will cover them now," she said and hung up.

Shortly after her call, Greg called in the facility administrator for a bedside chat with his father. The two men were angry. "Why did Dr. Silber cut off so many medications, when they might have been a big help?" Greg demanded to know.

After much dispute, I resumed the medications. Greg's health status remained the same. Only now the state, not the Farmer family, paid his pharmacy bill.

Greg became depressed. He would have benefited from psychological counseling. Medicaid, however, would pay only for a psychiatrist, who prescribed an antidepressant. He would not see Greg again for a month (all that insurance would allow) and then only for a brief visit.

Three weeks passed. Greg was still depressed. He refused to take the antidepressant, just as he often refused other medication. More and more immobile, he developed bedsores. He refused to bathe, and the sores became worse. Though he grew feverish, he continued to refuse care.

State surveyors were due in soon to inspect the facility. Greg's condition would certainly be seen as a red flag. The administrator called in his family to make a choice: Either Greg was hospitalized to receive intravenous antibiotics, or he should go into hospice care.

Greg chose hospice. The family decided that it was time for him to "pass." All medications were stopped, and Greg once again grew feverish. One weekend his father called in the extended family and a priest to stand over his bed. It was time to die. Greg would not oblige them. Instead he hopped out of bed, got into his electric wheelchair with the help of staff, and went outside to smoke a cigarette.

The following week representatives from hospice met with Greg and his family.

"Greg is getting better," they said, of his own accord. "He has the willpower to live." Hospice care stopped.

For about nine months, Greg remained stable. Then, once again, he became febrile and septic. This time he did not want hospitalization. "I'm ready to kick," he said.

A staff member called Greg's father. He and his daughter were leaving shortly on a Caribbean cruise. Death was not convenient now. His father sent Greg to the hospital, where he was treated with IV antibiotics and had skin flap surgery for his decubiti (costs covered by insurance).

Upon return from vacation, the family decided to take Greg home. He was ecstatic. Going home had never been mentioned as an option before. "I can't wait to get out of this stinking hellhole," he kept repeating. Mixed with venom was real elation.

There was still time left in his life for more bitterness, however. What at first glance had seemed an honest effort to care for Greg turned out to be the means to a financial end. Apparently, the family discovered that Greg had a pension (one hundred and twenty-five dollars a month) that he could draw on, provided that he was cared for at home.

Perhaps his sister told him the truth? In any case, Greg found out the real reason why his dad wanted to take him home. Once again, he did not oblige. He managed to die a few weeks later and never did go home.

A month after his death, I received a call from Greg's dad.

"Were you aware that Greg took a fall a few days before he died?"

"Yes," I said. "I was aware of that."

"Well, it's not listed on his death certificate."

"Why should it be?" I asked.

"Are you prepared to rule out negligence as a cause of death?

"Yes, I am," I said, stunned to hear him suggest otherwise.

"Well, we aren't." Mr. Farmer hung up on me.

Greg's family had worked every angle they could in the health care management system. His dad and his sister might be seen to represent still another category—the manipulative or predatory family. For its part, the facility protected its own needs just as well as the family had always protected theirs. Greg's care plan was always "appropriate" and "correct" throughout his stay. Greg's dad was not able to make good on his threat to sue.

In the two previous family sagas, we have seen quite a bit of dysfunction. Yet many times an elder ages and dies surrounded by a relatively normal, emotionally healthy family. Even then, the process is not a static one. The way in which the elder's care is managed may vary over time, depending on the family's hopes and goals and the care team's input at each juncture in the resident's life.

Ideal Evolution

Say, for example, that it is a family's hope that their ailing "Papa"—or "Poppy"—will regain his health to some degree. The family opts for skilled care within the nursing home setting.

Papa—The Business Model

Their father undergoes physical examination and then occupational, speech, and diagnostic testing. He sees medical specialists and takes advantage of every appropriate hospital service.

The day arrives, however, when the man's insurance will no longer pay for skilled care and will no longer authorize therapy services or specialized diagnostic testing. A care conference is held between the facility staff and the family. The administrator explains the situation.

"For your father to continue to receive therapy, you will have to pay out-of-pocket."

"Is it helping him a lot?" The man's eldest son asks.

"Not so much," one therapist answers and the others agree, with a nod of their heads.

"Then let's stop it," the eldest son says.

"We would be willing to pay for therapy if, at some point, it was decided that he could benefit from it," one of the daughters joins in to say.

The other family members agree with everything that has been said, again with a nod of their heads.

Papa—The Scientific Model

Papa's care undergoes a change. Whereas it used to be based on the business or insurance model, now it is based on scientific or medical care. Under the new plan, his care shifts from skilled to intermediate. Instead of therapy, he undertakes a daily physical fitness regimen with the help of a certified nurse assistant. He receives all of his medications, and sees his neurologist on occasion. For some time, he lives quite well. He begins to walk a bit.

Then after a few months, he develops a urinary infection, which is treated successfully. Overall, however, his health is not much better, despite all of the efforts he and the staff have made. He eats little and is losing weight. Soon he is no longer able to walk. A speech therapist's evaluation reveals that the man is not eating because he is unable to swallow. This incapacity often occurs in the final stages of dementia. He can no longer safely eat on his own, the therapist concludes. If he continues to do so, he will be at risk for aspiration pneumonia. (In other words, if he swallowed incorrectly, food could enter the lung instead of the stomach, with the possibility that he could develop an infection.) A feeding tube is suggested as an alternative means of feeding.

Once again, the staff and the family hold a care conference.

"We don't want a feeding tube," the eldest son says. "Poppy should eat as he pleases."

"Are you aware of the risks of aspiration?" the social worker asks.

The family members nod their collective heads.

As his dad's legal guardian, the eldest son signs a set of papers to affirm that the facility would not be held liable, should something "bad" happen as the result of "Poppy" eating as he pleases.

"We should stop some of his sedating medications," the doctor suggests. "That way, he might be more alert and eat better."

Hospice is discussed, but the family does not want this option.

Papa—The Ethical Model

The form of care shifts again, this time from the scientific to the ethical model. Though not in hospice, Poppy does eats what he wants, and his sedatives are discontinued. For a time, he perks up noticeably. A few months later, however, he develops another urinary tract infection. The family does not want him hospitalized. He is treated at the facility with intravenous fluids and antibiotics. Although he improves somewhat, he continues to be weak. He is no longer able to eat enough to sustain himself. He is uncomfortable. He needs more attention, and he needs to be repositioned to avoid bedsores.

Another care conference is scheduled. This time the family members agree to hospice, and the management of their father's care changes accordingly.

Papa—The Social Model

Under a social model, the man is made comfortable. He receives extra attention. Under hospice care, all of the special medical needs that contribute to his comfort are paid for by insurance. Meanwhile, his family members are educated and counseled as to how to cope when Poppy dies peacefully four months later.

Poppy's treatment evolved over the course of his last year of life. Together the facility staff and the family made use of all of the models of care designed to help patients in a variety of circumstances, and they used each one of them appropriately.

- **Stage One**: Hope for recovery (Business Model)—used all possible resources, particularly insurance
- **Stage Two**: Quiet period (Care Plan—Scientific Model)—made judicious use of medical and technological resources
- **Stage Three**: Possible dying (Ethical Model)—let nature take its course
- **Stage Four**: Prolonged dying process (Hospice)—actively managed dying with plenty of palliative care

13

Love, Beer, Sex, Drums

Among the nursing home population are those who are there for only a short time—people who stay anywhere from a few days to several months after an elective procedure or acute illness. After medical care and therapy, such residents generally return home and do well. Many become quite active and regain their independence after discharge.

Short-term rehabilitative stays are a great source of income to the long-term care facility. From a physician's perspective, however, there is a great legal risk associated with seeing a person only once or twice. In fact, the probability of some form of punitive action is high enough that doctors have grown reluctant to care for such residents. Likewise, it is the high risk associated with short-term residents that has led some insurers to deny liability coverage altogether to physicians who practice in long-term care facilities.

The risk arises out of the very lack of a relationship between the physician and the patient. The patient sees the physician once or twice for an acute condition (say, hip replacement), but the physician is held responsible for the problems associated with long-term, pre-existing conditions, such as diabetes or coronary disease, that have not been adequately managed. Longstanding anger and discontent can also factor into the situation and cause the resident or his family to look for someone to blame in a crisis. It does not help that the nursing home is often thought of as a place of mistrust, incompetence, and abuse.

Despite the risks, I do continue to see short-term residents. I may only see such residents once, if they stay for less than two weeks. Sometimes, however, they stay long enough for us to get to know one another.

ᦂ

A Recuperative Romance
Eva Weisman was among those whom I grew to know. At seventy, Eva had many health problems, including breast cancer and coronary

disease. After a fall, which led to surgery and an elective hip-joint replacement, she came to Sweet Penny Tree for rehabilitation. She was already familiar with the facility, not as a resident but as a family caregiver. Her younger sister, Rachel, had resided there, on and off, over the past several years for respite as well as for rehabilitation after acute illnesses. While Eva recuperated from her surgery at Sweet Penny Tree, Rachel stayed there, too, in a separate room, as she needed round-the-clock care and, in Eva's absence, there would be no one to look after her at home.

Eva benefited from rehabilitation. Her surgery had reduced her chronic pain significantly. Then therapy helped to strengthen her muscles. In a few weeks, she was in better physical health that she had been in many years. She remained in the facility for about a month and a half. During her stay, I saw her numerous times, and it became clear that she was depressed. Her low emotional state dated to her husband's death five years ago. I prescribed a mild antidepressant and talked to her about her loss.

When Eva's daughter came in one day to visit her, she pulled me aside in the hall to thank me.

"I'm so glad you put her on an antidepressant," she said. "My mom's so strong otherwise. Dad died a while ago. She really needs to get on with her life."

Overnight Eva became quite the socialite. In fact, the change occurred too quickly to ascribe it to her treatment for depression. An antidepressant requires a week or two to take effect. Within days of prescribing it, Eva was happy-go-lucky. The source of her joy lay elsewhere. For the first time in a long time, Eva was free from all the duties and obligations involved in taking care of Rachel. Clearly the two sisters were devoted to one another. Still, Rachel depended on Eva much like a very young child. Eva bathed and fed her, monitored her medications, and drove her everywhere. Instead of an endless round of chores, Eva could now play cards, watch a movie, or just sit and talk to other people over coffee. At some point, she renewed her old acquaintance with one of the volunteers, whom she had first met several years ago and saw again from time to time whenever Rachel returned to the facility for therapy. Chad was a widower. Now Eva had time to get to know him better. The two grew quite friendly and planned to have lunch together after her discharge.

As Eva prepared to leave the facility, the care team scheduled a conference. Such a discussion is routine and can include the resident's family and friends. Mrs. Weisman and her daughter, Melanie, attended, as did her sister, Rachel. In addition, Eva asked Chad to be present.

The care team reported excellent progress and suggested that Eva arrange for some help in taking care of Rachel. There was not much else to say. Medically, she was doing wonderfully, and there were no other issues.

Much to the care team's approval, Eva would be returning to Sweet Penny Tree as a volunteer. Her sister could come with her and do some outpatient therapy. Chad spoke up then and offered to sit with Rachel occasionally. For her part, Eva praised us for helping her out of depression. The care team applauded. Here was a success story, amid so much disability and illness.

Not everyone was pleased with the changes in Eva, as I discovered a few weeks later. Though she had not said a word during her mother's discharge conference, Melanie had plenty to say afterward when she called key members of the care team to express her displeasure.

Had her mother gone wild? How could Eva leave Rachel with anyone, let alone Chad? Dating at their age was simply ridiculous.

When the care team came to Eva's defense, Melanie called me.

"I'd like to discuss my mother's situation with you," she told me.

"I'll need her permission to do that," I reminded her.

"I don't want to talk about her medical condition," she snapped. "It's that man I'm calling about. The one who volunteers up at Sweet Penny Tree. He played up to Mom when she was in there. Now he's using her. I'm terribly upset to see her manipulated."

I made every effort to soothe. Still, I had to tell her the truth: "Your mother's private life is really out of my hands."

A few days later, Melanie called again.

"I've had a chance to think about it," she told me. "And I can see a number of possible explanations."

Maybe some of her medications were causing her mother's odd behavior. Maybe she was developing dementia. Or maybe her breast cancer metastasized to her brain.

"Can you order a CT scan of her brain?"

"That wouldn't be appropriate," I responded, but I wanted to offer her some reassurance if I possibly could. "You know, Melanie, nothing has changed in your mother's medications other than my adding an antidepressant. Many women her age seek male companionship. There's nothing abnormal about that."

For Chad and Eva, events moved quickly. Life was short, and the couple yearned to make the most of it. They were "old" and had the benefit of experience.

They announced their engagement to be married. They set a date and had their future all planned. After their wedding, they would move to a new apartment, one large enough to accommodate Rachel, who would live with them.

Melanie was not pleased. She continued to complain that her mother did not know what she was doing and was being used. Perhaps it was her displeasure that led Eva and her fiancée to prepare an extensive prenuptial agreement. Their respective children would lose nothing as a consequence of the marriage.

The wedding was as elegant as it was moving. I and a number of the staff from Sweet Penny Tree attended. Melanie, however, did not. She, who had once urged me to treat her mother for depression, remained disgusted with what she continued to view as "childish antics."

Not long after the marriage, Rachel became gravely ill. She went to live again at Sweet Penny Tree, where Eva continued to attend to her. In fact, she and her new husband visited daily. Several months later, Rachel died. She never became well enough to return to the newlyweds' home. The marriage was a good one. Eva and Chad continued to enjoy what each termed "the happiest time in my life." Rachel was sorely missed, of course—and so, sadly, was Melanie.

A Ladies' Man

Marc Scavino was seventy-five when he came to live at the Apple Lane nursing facility after an acute illness and hospitalization. He suffered from several chronic physical problems—cardiac disease, lung disease, and vascular disease. He also had a diagnosis of lung cancer, which he did not want treated. The consequences were quite severe. His heart problems caused swelling in his legs. Apart from cancer, he had trouble breathing after many years of smoking.

When he first arrived, he had a wound on his foot that needed care and antibiotics. He needed physical therapy to help him regain some of his strength. After some time Mr. Scavino's foot healed. The staff recommended physical therapy, but he was poorly motivated. For every order his doctor wrote for therapy, she wrote another to cancel it. He never did walk again without assistance. He remained in long-term care, partly because of that disability and partly because he had no place else to go.

I saw many residents at Apple Lane, but Marc was not among them until his payer source changed, and the physician initially assigned to him refused to follow him. As his doctor, I saw Marc once a month, but in fact I saw him often. He tended to stand out with his long, gray mane of hair. As I entered the building, there he would be, working on a crossword puzzle or reading the sports section. I would stop and ask how the local teams were doing. He would ask about my kids. A ladies' man, he would remark that he wished I were not married.

I could not cure Marc. However, there were some treatments that I could offer him to make him more comfortable and perhaps prolong his life and independence. At first he would agree to take the prescribed medication, but then refuse to, shortly after he got his first pill, stating that there were too many side effects. This reaction was a recurrent one, and I had extensive conversations with him to try and convince him that side effects were rarely dramatic.

Despite his refusal of medications, he was still "full code," that is, he wanted all advanced life support when on the verge of death. His choices were difficult to work with, but I respected his right to make them and did my best.

Marc's mental capacities were not compromised, and he often spoke of his dreams. He dreamt that he could walk on his own again, out in the fresh air. He dreamt of going back into construction work and watching football with his pals. However, there was always a reason why his dreams could not come true. The therapy was poor. The staff did not care about him.

He had friends in the facility and was close to some of the staff at Apple Lane, but he expressed a strong preference for the north side of town, where he used to hang out at the veterans' headquarters. As became clear after a few conversations, he was also a bit racist and complained about the large number of black residents and staff in the facility, although, ironically, they numbered among his friends.

One day the administrator called me in to say that Mr. Scavino was going to transfer to another facility, Drury-Campbell, near the VFW.

On the point of departure, Marc approached me himself and asked if I would take care of him at his new facility. I agreed to, although I had no other patients there. Initially, I also felt it somewhat burdensome to travel to the north side of the city to see just one person. Over time, however, my feelings changed.

Though a proud and guarded man, Marc savored every bit of human interaction he could get. He told me a new story every time I visited him. When employed, he had worked at odd jobs and in construction. He did what he wanted and had little interest in his wife and children when he was young. He did not appear to regret this neglect, though he was divorced now, and no one came to visit him.

"I have a family," he often said, and pointed to any staff member who happened to be in his vicinity.

Pretty soon I realized that Marc only pretended to dislike long-term care. In fact, he knew he was nearing the end of his life, and he did not want to be alone.

Beer on Doctor's Orders

Gradually, I found out more and more about him. He was unable to walk but wanted independence. He wanted therapy but was afraid that, if he failed, he would have to face the fact that he would never walk again.

He did want a beer or two a day. Was that okay?

Sure, I told him. No problem. I wrote an order for the staff to permit him to have up to two beers a night. Although he would not accept medications from me, he would "medicate" himself in his own way. Because he had no one else to do so, he depended on the staff to buy him a six-pack.

One month when I came to see him, he was very upset and asked to speak to me privately.

The social worker had confiscated his beer. In a departure from his usual routine, he had saved up some cans for an upcoming baseball game. Apparently, his small stockpile had caused a commotion in the facility and led to the social worker's raid.

"I had no idea," I told him. "No one on staff told me."

Marc did not seem surprised, although the social worker had claimed to him that I had been informed.

I rewrote the order. Now he could have up to fourteen beers a week and could drink them whenever he wanted.

After the beer raid, Marc opened up a little more. He told me that he spent most of his days in the hallway, listening to what was going on, but not saying much. He told me about squabbles among the staff and about their love affairs. I listened but said nothing. Though Marc never admitted to any regrets about his transfer to Drury-Campbell, he was often at odds with the staff members there, who were not as kind to him as they had been at Apple Lane, nor were they as tolerant of a point of view that differed from their own.

He fought, for example, to sleep at night in his chair. He had always slept in a chair, he explained, ever since he was a young adult.

The care team did not approve. A bed was the only place to sleep. A care plan was developed to get Mr. Scavino out of the chair and into the bed.

He continued to protest.

One day his chair was gone from his room. Upset, he called the state hotline. The chair reappeared almost as soon as it disappeared. Supposedly, the staff had sent it out to be cleaned.

A Right to Viagra

Despite his tense relations with many members of the staff, Marc had grown close to some of his fellow residents, who, as it happened, included several attractive women. Thus far, his relationships with these women were strictly platonic, he told me, but he hoped for more.

"I may have the body of an old man," he confided, "but my mind is still young and virile." He was seventy-six at the time. "How about Viagra, Doctor? Could you give me a prescription?"

I had no reason not to oblige him. "Only the facility won't pay," I warned him.

"That's okay," he said. "I'll pay for it myself."

Even then, his use of the drug would be anything but smooth. He would have to ask the nurses for a pill at the point that he needed it. Regulations forbid nursing home residents from possessing their own medications, which must be administered by the staff.

Sexual expression is a resident's right. However, some facilities are more accepting of sex than others. At Drury-Campbell, the nursing supervisor made it crystal clear that she did not want to administer Viagra to Mr. Scavino. She asked me to discontinue my order.

Of course, it was true that Mr. Scavino's use for Viagra remained theoretical. He was not involved in a sexual relationship. Furthermore, there was no guarantee that Viagra would have been effective, even if he had been. Still, I refused to cancel the order.

"Mr. Scavino has the right to try this drug, if he wants it," I said.

For a time, the issue lay dormant. Later, when Marc again expressed some serious interest in taking Viagra, the supervisor and her staff urged him to switch doctors. He did not follow their advice, though he never did fill his prescription.

Viagra aside, I did continue to offer him some treatments for his heart condition and occasional episodes of pneumonia. Typically, he would not take any medicine for long. He went to the hospital a few times for breathing problems. Despite his desire for no treatment, Marc continued to be full code.

On several occasions, I asked why.

"I don't trust people around here," he answered, "especially not Janice." She was the social worker, who had confiscated his beer and the very staff member assigned to discuss advanced directives with the residents.

"I don't want to depend on the staff," he added. "They do what's in their interests, not mine."

I made no comment. I had little to do with the staff. I had a good patient load and was not actively pursuing new business. I came to the facility with the purpose of following Marc and only Marc. With so little interaction, it was not surprising that I had developed so little rapport with the staff. Besides, Marc was not well liked. Perhaps this dislike extended to me? Of course many staff members disapproved of some of my decisions regarding his care. They were not pleased that I allowed him beer and Viagra, and they were not pleased that I allowed him to refuse other medications. They treated me with a mixture of distrust and animosity.

When Marc began to have more health problems, he asked to see me, but, as we discovered, I did not always receive his messages. I gave him my business card, although he had no phone to call me in his room. When I did see him, I prescribed medicine. As usual, he would take it for a few days and then stop because of supposed side effects. He declined faster than if he had followed medical advice. Despite refusing treatment, he would never sign "do not resuscitate" papers. He remained an enigma to the end: He refused care when offered but refused to state that he did not want it.

Even with severe pneumonia and congestive heart failure, he refused antibiotics and other curative medications. He was too weak to resist the male nurse who put him into bed one night. Hours later, however, he awoke and attempted to walk over to his beloved armchair, where he preferred to sleep. On the way there, he fell to the floor, unconscious.

The staff sent him to the hospital. He did not return. He died on a ventilator with a feeding tube inserted. I was not informed until several weeks after the fact. No one on staff called me the night of Marc's fall.

Trips to the emergency room often occurred after hours, when the staff could say that the physician on call, namely, a colleague covering for me, ordered the transfer. In fact, the staff probably transferred him without any physician's order.

Two years later, the other physicians in my practice became interested in building up business. As it happened, one of them paid a call on the facility where Marc had lived out his last days. She met with the administrator (who didn't know me, having come to the facility after I had left). They discussed the idea of a doctor from our organization following the residents at the facility who were discharged from our hospitals.

"Not Dr. Silber," the administrator said, apparently quite categorically. "I won't allow her to follow residents in this facility."

"Why not?" my colleague asked.

The facility did not like my documentation, or rather, the lack thereof.

Many times the staff at Drury-Campbell had failed to relay messages to me from Marc—lapses that he often mentioned, though ones he seemed to take in stride—or else I received word in a less than timely manner. I always responded quickly whenever I did hear from the staff, however, and Marc offered no complaints regarding my care. In fact, he had gone out of his way to keep me as a physician over the years. Now, however, the situation had come back to bite. Somehow lapses on the part of the staff were attributed to me. Somehow the administrator came to believe that I had not answered my calls. Somehow beer and Viagra may have had something to do with it.

The Music Maker

Frank Olympia came to live at Fern Oakes when he was about forty-five. For more than a decade, he had been enduring the progressively degenerative effects of multiple sclerosis. If the disease was progressing, Frank was not. He came to long-term care after a suicide attempt and a psychiatric hospitalization. Still despondent, he arrived with little hope, though he could move around in a wheelchair and remained mentally alert.

Before his disease had overtaken him, he had led a colorful life. As a drummer in a heavy metal band, he had traveled the world and had seen most everything. He had lived life to the fullest. Now that his world had shrunk so drastically, he spent most of his days sleeping, listening to music, watching videos, and smoking cigarettes—preferably ones made of marijuana when he could pay to buy some. Unlike the Drury-Campbell facility, Fern Oakes took a laissez-faire attitude toward resident lifestyles. The administration tended to look the other way, rather than confront illicit activities.

Still handsome, Frank was quick to take up with several young women in the facility. No one interfered with his romances. In fact, the staff noticed that, once he had a girlfriend, he settled down and complied more with his care plan and took his medications regularly.

Over the months that followed, Frank did what he could to help himself. After some psychotherapeutic counseling, he came to terms with his life and accepted the fact that he did indeed have a progressive disease. It was unlikely that he would ever live on his own again, let alone roam the world freely the way he used to do.

Meanwhile, the physical therapy and other medical care that he received in the facility prolonged his life and continued to strengthen him and make him more independent. He had disabilities, yes, but he relearned how to do many things for himself. If he did not engage much in the collective life of the facility, neither did he ask for much in return.

After he had been in the facility for six months, he did begin to show renewed signs of discontent and depression, though never to the degree that had preceded his attempted suicide.

"I sure haven't accomplished much," he told me one day. "And that bothers me."

"You've traveled more than anyone I know," I said.

"Yeah, but that was just fun and games. It doesn't add up."

I saw his point and wondered what he might do.

The physical therapist on staff spotted Frank's dissatisfaction, too. He suggested that Frank pick up the guitar again. If nothing else, the effort might help build upper body strength and ward off a breakdown in coordination.

So Frank began to pluck an electric guitar. Fern Oakes was elaborate enough to have a sound-proof room, where he could practice without disturbing anyone. Little by little, however, a few of the residents would slip into the chairs at the back to listen to Frank play. Though he had lost some of his motor skills, he still sounded like what he had once been—a professional musician. Instinctively, he responded to his new environment. He moved away from heavy metal in favor of soulful ballads by Pat Metheny.

The physical therapist, who had suggested that he play, was thrilled. Impressed with Frank's abilities, he consulted with a music therapist, who did some part-time work at Fern Oakes. Together they proposed a plan and took it to Frank. Would he be willing to form a band in the facility?

Frank was willing, though it would take him years to teach enough residents to play passably well. Even then, he was under no illusions. "We're approaching the musical level of an elementary school without the freshness that kids would bring to the sound," he once remarked.

Yet the effort did everyone good. Frank surprised himself. He had no idea that he could teach. He had no inkling that showing frail and elderly men and women how to play the drums would feed his soul.

Frank had become an asset to the facility and to the other residents. As he gave to others, he derived a kind of pleasure that he had never experienced.

"Believe it or not," he said to me one day after band practice, "I think I've accomplished something—though it's sure not 'Black Sabbath.'"

At about this time, Frank's love life took a serious turn. He and Audrey, one of his night nurses, grew quite close.

As relaxed as Fern Oakes was, certain standards still applied. Audrey was given a choice: Either she stopped dating Frank, or she should find a job elsewhere. Without hesitation, she quit Fern Oakes and went to work at another facility. The staff did not have to wait long to find out if the two would remain an item. Shortly after Audrey left Fern Oakes, Frank began to spend the night at her home several times a month. Without comment, the nurse on duty provided him a pass to do so. Even after Frank married Audrey and left Fern Oakes for good, he remained the facility's volunteer band leader and instructor for many years.

14

Odd Men Out

It is said that social life in a nursing home is a lot like social life in high school. Though a debatable remark, it is true that the population is made up of quite a few resident cliques. They include elders with dementia and behavioral problems, young people with traumatic brain injury and impulsive behaviors, as well as the chronically mentally and physically ill who have a prison history and no place to go after parole or discharge.

Young and Heavy

Justin Williamson was introduced earlier as an example of a newcomer to long-term care—the morbidly obese or "bariatric" patient—who has begun to show up more often in facilities in recent years. Weighing more than five hundred pounds, all of Justin's physical problems stemmed directly from his physical condition. In addition to diabetes and hypertension, he had developed severe osteoarthritis and was unable to walk by the time that he entered the Sonoma Ranch facility. Congestive heart failure caused massive swelling in his lower extremities. In turn, this swelling caused weeping of fluid from his skin and open sores to develop. His anatomy was so contorted that he was unable to urinate on his own.

Before coming to the facility, Justin had lived with his mother who had washed her son, something that he was unable to do himself. She took him to the toilet, as he was unable to wipe himself. When she became too ill to continue, he developed an infection in his legs, the result of poor hygiene. Thus her own illness prompted his move into long-term care.

Justin was so obese that it interfered with his breathing. He had developed sleep apnea, a respiratory obstruction that he coped with by sleeping in a sitting position at night. He was supposed to use a special machine to help him breathe but refused it. Occasionally, his oxygen level dropped so low that he would turn blue and faint. Oxygen, fortunately, would quickly bring him back to consciousness.

As mentioned earlier, Justin was not the only bariatric patient in the facility. He became friendly with two other residents who were in a similar physical state and spent most of his days watching television with them. In some ways, the bonds that he developed with these men were good for Justin. Obesity had affected his psychological growth. Before he came to Sonoma Ranch, he had had no relationships outside his family. His physical limitations prevented him from holding a job, and he had engaged in very few of the activities typical of young people his age. Obese since childhood, Justin had never participated in activities typical of children, either.

Unable to fit into a car or bus, he was practically trapped at home. He and his mother waited until he became sick enough to call 911. Then the paramedics would make arrangements to transport him to the hospital. On his last trip to the hospital before he arrived at Sonoma Ranch, the fire department had to be called to break down a doorway so that the paramedics could get him out of the house.

Justin had the emotional development of a five year old. He cried when he did not get what he wanted. Though his doctors had prescribed an array of medications, he tended to take only those for pain and to skip the rest. Months after he arrived at Sonoma Ranch, the staff still bribed him, usually with food or cigarettes, to get him to take his pills.

His sister, June, continued to cook for him. Whenever she visited the facility, she would unpack a basket full of delicious meals and snacks. June's ritualized presentation of home-cooked food and the appreciative smack of Justin's lips in return was as close to human intimacy as these two had ever come.

The facility afforded Justin a number of ways to change his life. His major breakthrough, however, was to make friends with the two aforementioned bariatric patients, who lived at Sonoma Ranch at the time. The unfortunate consequence of this otherwise happy development was the reinforcement of self-destructive habits, which the three men enjoyed in each other's company, including smoking, eating to excess, and remaining sedentary for hours at a time in front of one of the facility's several large television sets. Now and then, Justin truly did try to cut back on pizza and cigarettes, but his attempts were short-lived. As genuine as his intentions were, he had little stamina, and the staff was too busy to offer him the consistent support he needed to prevail. As it was, he continued to place high demands on the staff's time and would cry if he did not receive immediate attention.

A year after he had come to live at Sonoma Ranch, Justin was rushed to the hospital. A nurse had found him in the staff lounge, where he had been sneaking a cigarette and then turned blue. Once hospitalized, he did not survive. Justin died on a ventilator when he was thirty-eight.

When Success Is a Problem

Herschel White was forty-five when he entered long-term care. Unable to move or care for himself, he had undergone several unsuccessful knee replacements. Within a year of his arrival at Apple Lane, however, he had made an impressive recovery. Additional surgery, good nursing, physical therapy, and medical care had combined to work wonders. Herschel began to walk to nearby meetings of Alcoholics Anonymous and from there to the shopping mall. Before long, he was covering distances of two to three miles a day and spending more time outside than inside the facility. I began to wean him off pain medication, which he no longer needed, and directed the staff to begin planning his discharge from long-term care.

The social worker counseled him on prospective job training programs and how he might go about finding an apartment. It was shortly afterward that Herschel began to change. He called the state hotline to complain: I was withholding medication, which was causing him pain, and the nursing staff was negligent. He could not substantiate his complaints. In fact, he no longer needed medical or nursing care. The consensus was unanimous and one with which the state found no fault.

Shortly after his talk with the social worker, Herschel called the staff in one night. He stated that, as he lay in bed, an insect had emerged from his roommate's skin and had bit him. When I asked him where, he pointed to his upper thigh, where I did find an unusual puncture wound. I treated him with antibiotics, but his wound grew in size. The wound care nurse evaluated him but was at a loss. Herschel, meanwhile, continued to feel strong enough to go out daily on his long walks. One day he went out and never returned.

The administrator notified the police, but his whereabouts remained a mystery.

A year later, I received a registered letter in the mail. I opened the envelope to read that I was being sued, along with the facility. At the bottom of the page, there was his name. Herschel White was the plaintiff in the lawsuit against us.

He claimed that we had mismanaged his pain and caused him such duress that he left the facility. With nowhere to go, he became homeless. His knee became infected again, as he slept outside most of the time. He was admitted to the hospital, and his leg was amputated for gangrene.

How sad, I thought, despite the lawsuit. Herschel had never wanted to leave the facility, where he could count on a warm room and hot meals, and yet remain free to move about town during the day. His bizarre attempt to stay at the facility signaled his desperation. Clearly he had punctured himself, though he had blamed the self-inflicted skin wound on his roommate, an elderly male with dementia.

Unbending Fury

Like Justin Williamson, Greg Farmer was introduced earlier in these pages. He had come to the nursing facility when he was twenty-nine, after a spinal cord injury caused by a dive into an empty pool. Paralyzed from the neck down, he underwent multiple surgeries and extensive rehabilitation but was never able to use his legs again, though he did regain some upper extremity movement.

During his recovery, his girlfriend gave birth to a son. Initially, she and the baby would come and visit him often, but things changed over time. Greg became more and more angry. He abused the staff, and he refused care. Consequently, he developed a wound so large that he required surgery and an amputation of part of his leg. He also needed a colostomy and a supra-pubic catheter from his bladder.

After extensive hospitalization, however, he was doing fairly well by the time he returned to the facility. Only by then he had broken off communication with his girlfriend entirely. (His father and sister visited him rarely.) The one person whom he continued to see regularly was his stepfather, a Mr. Burns, who saw to it that Greg had a carton or two of cigarettes.

Five or six years after Greg's accident, Mr. Burns was diagnosed with terminal lung cancer. He died a month or so later. Greg was left to depend on the staff members, whom he had abused so consistently, as his primary source of human contact. Although his insurance would not pay for psychotherapy, he did receive some help after the staff persuaded a psychologist to see Greg free of charge. These counseling sessions did make a remarkable difference. Greg did become a bit more content and likeable. He did develop a few friends in the facility. In a momentous step, he called his girlfriend and apologized for his behavior. His son, who was then about five, began to visit him every month or so.

Beauty in Defiance

Tobias Keller was in his early thirties when I first met him. Diabetic since he was a child, he had an impressive handle on how to take care of himself and endure. Unlike so many in his situation, Toby had not refused care, which allowed him to survive his genetic illness past the age of thirty, something that would have been impossible just a few decades before.

For as long as he could, he had lived alone in an apartment and had found ways to rely on public insurance and services to remain self-sufficient. He managed his financial affairs and the laborious task of filing insurance claims. He did his own taxes. All the same, most of his time was given over to extensive treatments for his poor health and disabilities. His kidneys had failed. To filter his blood, he underwent dialysis up to six hours a day, three times a week.

He came to the Wentworth nursing facility after the amputation of his left leg. For five years, he shuttled back and forth between the hospital and the long-term care facility. Blood transfusions and medical procedures filled his days for the rest of his thirties. He spent his thirty-fifth birthday at Wentworth as well as his fortieth. In the end, he lost his second leg.

After the amputation, I expected to help Toby deal with bitterness and despair. What did he have to look forward to—loss of his eyesight?

Through scientific advances, we prolong the existence of people like him, I thought, but we have failed to create a real "place" for them. It was impossible for Toby to lead a normal life—to hold a job, marry, or have children. His father had died, and his mother was in poor health. His sister also had diabetes and likewise spent her time tethered to dialysis.

Remarkably, even mysteriously, Toby did not lose hope or courage. Though confined now to a wheelchair, he managed to return to his apartment and live there for nearly nine months. During that time, he found and used a subsidized cab service to take him to and from dialysis. In his few spare hours, he began to study computer science. Even after his declining health forced him to return to Wentworth, he never gave up on his academic goal. Surrounded by textbooks, he gave me a grin and told me that he hoped to earn a degree someday.

If he died too soon, he lived with a beautiful kind of bravery right up until the end.

Opting Out

I got to know Donald Jackson on paper before I actually saw him. Diagnosed with a rare form of skin cancer, Donald was a hospice patient in his late thirties when his caregivers called to ask Sweet Penny Tree to accept his request for admission to a long-term care facility. Shortly after their call, his medical charts arrived. The manager of admissions and the facility marketing representative asked me to review them and make sure that Mr. Jackson was admitted as quickly as possible. The facility was in need of admissions; many beds were empty at the time.

Eagerly, I agreed. I certainly wanted to please the facility administrators. As a brand new doctor, I also was in need of patients to build my practice. I began to read the massive documentation on Mr. Jackson that very afternoon. With so few patients, I could afford to be particularly careful in considering his medical history even in so short an amount of time. After reading every word, it struck me that something was just not right.

The diagnosis of cancer had been made ten years ago. Yet it was not cited again in his charts until three years ago, when he first enrolled in hospice. Subsequently, he skipped from one hospice program to another, staying in each for less than a year. As a hospice patient, he had agreed to nonaggressive treatment because of his terminal condition and therefore had not seen an oncologist for at least three years.

My interest was piqued by the absence in the charts of any indication that Mr. Jackson's cancer had progressed over the years.

I put a call into the oncologist who had made the diagnosis. After consulting his own medical records, he called me back to report that Mr. Jackson had long been cured of his cancer. Although a rare form of the disease, it was one that was easy to treat.

As I absorbed what the oncologist had told me, I began to put together a possible explanation for what I had read in the chart. In every hospice, he was prescribed medications for pain. It appeared to me that he had used his cancer diagnosis as a reason. By moving from one facility to another, he avoided questions. Then, too, hospice by its very nature tends not to inspire careful review of a patient's medical history—certainly not the kind that his charts had just undergone by an avid young doctor.

When I reported my findings to the manager of admissions and to the administrator, they quickly called the hospice caregiver to deny Mr. Jackson admission to Sweet Penny Tree. They did not want to fill an empty bed with what appeared to be a resourceful drug addict.

A weeks or so later, I headed into Malcolm Heights, another nursing facility where I had been hired as an attending physician. Who should be assigned to me but Donald Jackson. I was to manage his care. Obviously, no one at Malcolm Heights had devoted an afternoon to going over his chart.

As I already knew, Donald was thirty-seven and had spent a number of years in prison. He had had a rough childhood, filled with paternal abuse. Otherwise, his records showed no evidence of any family in his life. I never did find out what crime put him behind bars, but doing time had been hard on his health. For reasons unknown, his medical records showed that he had developed neurological problems while in prison, which had left him unable to walk. When I first began to see him, his body was so contorted that it was difficult even to move or to bathe him. He spent most of the day curled up in a fetal position.

As it turned out, he did not have a neurological illness. My first thought was to try physical and occupational therapy. Hospice might well be inappropriate, if he could regain mobility.

He refused. "It never helped me before, and it won't help me now."

He also refused to take the antidepressant prescribed for him at his last hospice facility.

"I'm not depressed," he insisted.

Although he showed no interest in me, I was interested in him. Why would a young man be satisfied with life in a nursing home and make no attempt to get better?

In time, I had my answer: Don knew what ailed him, and he was not looking for a cure. Sometime during his prison years, he had decided he was better off disabled than to try and survive there otherwise. He took to his bed and developed contractures so that he could not walk. Sickness brought relief from prison life. With little incentive to become better, he refused medical care. He refused physical therapy.

Once out of prison, he was stuck with the consequences of his long immobility. His muscles had atrophied, and his skin had broken down. He needed plastic surgery for his wounds. Although treatment options were available, he did not understand what positive consequences were, having experienced very few in his life. He continued to refuse care. Through the years, he had mastered one skill and that was how to manipulate the various social systems that he encountered. Though he had managed to survive, he had also hobbled himself. Now when he had a chance to regain his independence, he passed it by. He had a strong sense of mistrust— too strong to try to take a chance on a new life.

Donald remained in hospice within the framework of long-term care. He was content to lie inert in his bed, where, at the end of his life, he was nursed with some tenderness.

Crazy Way to Go

And what of Gilbert Pollick, an odd man out, if ever there was one? With his long history of chronic mental illness, he lived on for many years in the Apple Lane behavior unit, where he spent much of his time in his room, contemplating. His contemplations led to thoughts about his bowels, his penis, and, as mentioned earlier, a preoccupation with insomnia, though he routinely slept through the night. Known as a complainer without a cause, he was considered harmless—an annoyance and not a threat.

The threat appeared in the form of a second Gilbert, who came to live on the Apple Lane behavioral unit. At forty-seven, Gilbert Hue had a history of chronic pain, dating to an automobile accident twenty years earlier. Soon evident as well was his severe personality disorder, which apparently had gone untreated because of his denial and refusal of care.

One day at lunch another newcomer took Gilbert Pollick's usual seat at the table. The "old" Gilbert moved on to sit in a chair elsewhere. Unfortunately for him, the "new" Gilbert already considered the chair his own. The new Gilbert pinned the old Gilbert to the ground and urinated on him. Humiliated, the old Gilbert became reclusive, rightfully fearing ridicule from the other residents on the unit. He took his meals in his room and went out only to smoke.

For a few weeks, all was calm. Then one afternoon, Gilbert Hue spotted Gilbert Pollick outside in the courtyard, puffing on his usual after-lunch cigarette. He stepped out the door, and the two men quickly got into another altercation.

As later reported by a member of the staff who witnessed what happened, the new Gilbert directed a racial slur at the old Gilbert.

Incensed, Gilbert Pollick slapped the younger man hard across the face.

The staff member quickly intervened at that point. He appeared to resolve the situation, and no one was hurt.

Afterward, however, the administrator at Apple Lane called Gilbert Hue in to discuss what the facility could do to make his stay more comfortable: He was a new admission and needed to be treated well, so that he and his payer source would stay in the facility.

The following morning, a nurse found Gilbert Pollick strangled in his bed.

His death was a tremendous shock, to say the least. A little investigation on my part turned up the fact that Gilbert Hue had served time for murder.

Administrators at the corporate level, meanwhile, were quick to rule Gilbert Pollick's death as accidental. He had left behind no family or friends to question the determination.

Before the week was over, I was let go as Apple Lane's medical director.

"You've done nothing wrong," the administrator assured me, and, indeed, my letter of dismissal indicated satisfaction with my services. "It's just that you've been here a long time. Corporate thinks we need a fresh approach."

Still, Gilbert Hue remained on the behavior unit, where he remained a terrible risk to facility residents and staff.

15

After the Rounds — and Then Some

I arrive at Fern Oakes, the last facility that I will visit today. The yearly inspection is in full swing, though nothing about the place looks unusual, except for the official poster taped to each door, stating that a state survey is under way.

I find Nina Winger, the director of nursing. Understandably, she is too harried to offer me her usual warm smile of welcome. She does give me a list of things that I need to do while I am here.

The nurse who treats skin problems quit this morning. The job is a critical one.

"I begged her to please stay until state was gone," Nina tells me, "but she just got up and left."

I visit a long-time patient of mine, Nellie Bush, who has just fractured her hip. There was no documentation of her fall; that is, no one witnessed it. Her pain and the big bruise on her skin are the evidence. The administrator asks me to document the unavoidability of the fracture.

Nellie cannot tell me what happened. She has advanced dementia. Her sister, who has mild dementia, however, might know something. Mildred Bush is also a resident at the facility and her sister's advocate.

"Nellie has several problems today," Mildred tells me when I go in to see her. "She has pain, constipation, and is not eating well."

I tell her that I will prescribe something to make her sister more comfortable.

She nods. On my way out, she remarks, "I've never seen so many staff in the facility. They're here to impress the inspectors, isn't that right, Doctor?"

"It may be," I say and give her a smile. After all, I am the medical director—paid to support the facility. I better watch my tongue— even with a demented woman.

I see two more residents with no difficulties and leave the facility ahead of schedule.

At home an hour later, the phone rings. The Fern Oakes administrator is on the line, breathless. "There's an important document, Doctor, which should've been signed off months ago. You need to sign it right away. The nurses keep meaning to mention it to you, but they keep forgetting. We really need your cooperation."

"Have someone bring it by this afternoon," I tell him.

"I'm too busy to do that, what with the state inspectors in here."

I guess it is not so important after all.

Paper Trail

After a quick sandwich at my desk, the next part of my day is about to begin. I must document my visits and justify a treatment plan—or a lack thereof. (If a resident does not agree to what is recommended, I must document the fact as well.) In any case, I must record my time with each resident to receive compensation from the insurers. Payment is based more on actions than on the deliberative and decision-making processes that lead up to them. My lengthy conversation with Joe Scott, the AIDS patient at Apple Lane, for example, is essentially gratis. I will be compensated largely on the basis of how many changes I made in his medications and how many organ systems I addressed. If I make a change in his care plan and document it properly, I will get paid more. If I think that no change is in order, I have not "worked" hard enough and will be paid less.

Usually, I spend about five hours a day on documentation—about the same amount of time I spend seeing residents. I break up the documentation (which is both tedious and taxing) by answering mail and faxes.

I spend at least an hour a day on mail, which consists mostly of forms needing a signature. Orders that I give over the phone are subsequently written down and mailed to me. Under state law, I must sign these orders and return them to the proper facilities within forty-eight hours of receipt.

Faxes are another daily feature. Typically, I get about one hundred a day and sort them into several categories. Today I receive thirty pharmacy signatures for narcotics; forty normal and abnormal labs for my review; ten incident (e.g., fall with no injury) and similar reports; ten specific requests for information by the end of the day; five requests for critical information that require follow-up phone calls by the end of the day; and five dense reports, which require complex decision making.

I finish my documentation. I finish my mail. I have received one handwritten note from a family member, thanking me for taking care of her mom, who has just passed away. I have received one typewritten note, stating unhappiness with my care as a doctor at a certain facility. "Frankly I am appalled by such subhuman treatment," the writer signs off, though he offers no specifics. I do not recognize the resident's name, which is odd. I look her up on my computer; her name is not in my system. I call the facility. Sadie Green, I am told, is indeed seen by another physician. That doctor just received a similar note.

Two more faxes need to be addressed. Then my "official" day is done.

On Call

Some days never do feel "done," officially or otherwise. That sense is especially common when I am on call, as I was this past weekend. Sunday and Monday have blended into what feels like one day—a day that never ends.

Fielding phone calls after office hours is part of my job. As a member of a group of physicians, I am expected to take such calls one day a week and one weekend a month for all five of us physicians who make up the practice. Being on call on a weekday means returning calls to the practice from seven in the evening until eight the next morning. On weekends, being on call is a twenty-four-hour-a-day proposition, from nine in the morning one day through nine in the morning the next. The arrangement means each of us is free four out of five weekday evenings, as well as four out of five weekends.

When on call, we respond to reported changes in our residents' medical conditions that may require a physician's care. Other calls are a tad more mundane. To illustrate, here are some sample entries that I logged in during the last twenty-four-hour, Sunday-to-Monday period. I responded to each call as soon as I received it, usually within five minutes.

Sunday Morning

9:33 a.m.—I respond to an emergency call from the Ridgewood Home. I listen to the phone ring and ring. I wait five minutes and call again. Still no answer. I repeat the process, and this time the nurse picks up. A resident is having profuse rectal bleeding and looking pale. The vital signs (pulse, blood pressure, and temperature) are unstable. I tell the nurse to send the resident to the emergency room.

10:12 a.m. — A woman calls. She is the daughter of a resident whom I have cared for over many years. She has never called me before. This morning she tells me that she has done some research on the Internet and would like certain tests done on her mom. I suggest other testing that may be more appropriate.

The daughter is not happy. She insists that the evaluation that she discovered be done. "I've been looking into this for a week now. If you don't order the tests, I'll find another doctor who will."

I am tempted to tell her to look for another physician. Then I think of her mother, who made me a birthday card and mailed it to my home. I oblige without comment.

10:22 a.m. — A man and his sister are visiting their father, whom they think is acting strangely. They insist that he be sent to the emergency room. I ask the nurse on duty if the ER is warranted. She says no. I agree, nonetheless, to send the resident to the hospital. I have learned from experience not to question the inevitable. Once family members are dead-set on the ER, no amount of logic will change their minds.

11: 06 a.m. — An elderly male with prostate cancer is confused. I order some testing within the facility. His son calls to ask me whether his father should be sent to the emergency room. I give him my reasons for advising against the trip to the hospital. He confers with his wife and then comes back on the line to accept what I say.

11:12 a.m. — A hospice resident dies. I am called for an order to release the remains, as required by state law. I pronounce death over the telephone. A nurse cannot, even as she stands over the deathbed.

11:20 a.m. — A supervisor calls to say that one of the residents is growing more and more agitated. I assess the situation and relay some orders, but the supervisor says she cannot write them down. She needs to call me back after she finds a pencil.

11:26 a.m. — A resident with metastatic cancer is not doing well and needs an increase in pain medications.

11:54 a.m. — A resident's medication needs a change in dosage, in line with the day's laboratory data.

11:56 a.m.—A resident falls with no injury, which for regulatory reasons the nurse must report.

Sunday Afternoon

12:13 p.m.—A resident with nausea has developed a fever. The nurse asks for a Tylenol order.

12:20 p.m.—A staff member calls to say that a resident bit her. What should be done?

12:26 p.m.—A resident with diabetes has an increase in blood sugar after eating cake and ice cream at another resident's birthday party. I give an order to administer extra insulin and to recheck his blood sugar in a few hours.

1:06 p.m.—A resident has a urinary infection. When I call back, the nurse states that she has misplaced the relevant paperwork (information I need to put the resident on the appropriate antibiotic). She will call me when she is prepared to talk to me.

2:00 p.m.—I return a call from "Sharon." The receptionist states that no Sharon is working in the building. I explain that she just called me. Reluctantly, the receptionist agrees to page the name, though she says that I must be responding to a call from yesterday. Sharon is located. She reports some x-ray and lab results on several residents who are ill.

2:13 p.m.—A nurse calls about a clarification of an order I wrote earlier in the week. Apparently, the order has not been carried out. "Why have they waited until mid-day Sunday to call me," I ask. "I don't know," the nurse tells me, "I only work on Sundays."

2:27 p.m.—An end-stage Alzheimer's resident is dehydrated. Her family does not want her sent to the hospital but would like some intravenous fluids, if I think they would add to her comfort. I discuss options with the family, who are in the facility. They are grateful that I have taken the time to talk to them and help them to make a difficult decision.

2:29 p.m.—A nurse calls to ask me how to spell my name. She needs it for her records.

2:33 p.m.—State inspectors have arrived at Fern Oakes for their yearly review. The facility needs an order for an x-ray on a resident who fell a week ago.

3:09 p.m.—A resident of mine dies. She was ninety-nine. She went to temple with her family yesterday and had a good time. The nurse who called to tell me is distressed.

"She died—just like that." I can hear her snap her fingers. "I'm going to ask her family if they want an autopsy. I mean, what was the cause of death?"

"We will all die," I tell her, "even if we aren't on medications and have no disease."

3:20 p.m.—A nurse does not remember why she called me. She left her paperwork somewhere else. She will call me later, if she needs to.

3:33 p.m.—A nurse reports critical labs from Friday (more than forty-eight hours ago). I ask how the resident is doing. I cannot judge based on old data. She does not know, she says, and will call me back.

3:44 p.m.—I am paged. I call back. The nurse who called is on break. The covering nurse does not know what the other one wanted.

3:50 p.m. A resident was found smoking "weed" in her room because she has a headache. Do I have some medical remedy the nurse can offer her instead?

4:45 p.m.—The nurse who reported the Friday lab data calls back to say that the resident's vitals and condition are unchanged. I order repeat labs from Friday's "stat" and ask to be called (within an hour).

5:10 p.m.—A resident at Fern Oakes has complained to state inspectors that he does not like the antibiotic that he is on and wants a "stronger" one. Given his positive response to current treatment, I refuse a change until he is reassessed.

5:57 p.m.—I respond to a page from Ridgewood Manor. "This is Dr. Silber. I'm answering a call."

"Are you a family member?" the unidentified person who answers the phone asks. "What exactly are you calling about?"

"I am a physician, and I am calling regarding a resident."

"Well, there is no Dr. Silber in the building."

"I am Dr. Silber," I reply. "A nurse just called me."

She seems to understand now and puts me on hold. Five minutes later, she comes back on the line. "No one called you."

I ask her to re-page the nurse as I certainly have been called. I have it logged into my answering service network. Reluctantly, the woman complies. The nurse who called me is located. A resident has a bruise on her arm, which needs to be reported. I respond as graciously as I can.

Sunday Evening

6:00 p.m.—A hospice resident has died. The family from out of town is upset and would like to talk to the physician.

6:25 p.m.—I verify admission orders on a woman with dementia who is entering long-term care for a respite stay while the family is on vacation. The woman is anxious and tearful. Already she has fallen. At the same facility, a resident who is a known abuser of pain medications has returned from a day pass, glassy-eyed and lethargic. The staff reports that she was seen at the bus stop, drinking from a bottle concealed in a brown paper bag. Now that she is back, she is asking for her pain medications. What should the staff do?

6:30 p.m.—The nurse calls back, who was going to provide an update on Friday labs. She has found more recent lab results but has temporarily misplaced them. She will look for them and call me back in a minute.

6:45 p.m.—The nurse pages me with the misplaced labs. I call back and let the phone ring multiple times, but no one answers.

6:49 p.m.—The administrator calls from Fern Oakes, the facility where the state is doing an inspection. The resident that does not like the antibiotic is still refusing to take it. Apparently, he has looked up drugs on the Internet and wants a more expensive one. The director of nursing wants me to change the antibiotic, as the resident is making "trouble" with the surveyors. He is doing well with the current treatment, I repeat.

7:00 p.m.—A staff member calls me from Sweet Penny Lane. She has a favor to ask. Her son was in an auto accident yesterday and is very ill. She needs me to prescribe her something for her nerves for a few days. I oblige and call her pharmacy. I have known this person for some time and trust her. I do see some facility staff as patients.

7:20 p.m.—A resident is having hallucinations and is hitting staff. This is not a new behavior. A small dose of an antianxiety medication usually helps. What do I think?

7:30 p.m.—One of my residents with dementia states that oxygen makes her feel better. An order is needed.

7:44 p.m.—The floor nurse at Fern Oakes calls. The resident who insists he wants his antibiotics changed has announced that he is choosing another physician. I ask to speak to him.

"Why are you so adamant about changing antibiotics when you're doing so well?" I ask.

"Joey (one of the staff members) told me his mother did real poorly on it," he says. "That's why."

"Can you wait until tomorrow, and we can talk about this in person?"

He calms a bit and agrees.

7:49 p.m.—A resident fainted in the dining room and was a "full code"; 911 was dispatched.

7:55 p.m.—A nurse reports labs from today.

Sunday Night

8:10 p.m.—The emergency room calls: The resident who fainted in the dining room has expired. Am I willing to sign the death certificate?

8:15 p.m.—The nurse calls back for the fourth time about Friday's labs. I tell her that I returned her call earlier.

"Sorry," she says, "there is no receptionist on Sundays."

The "stat" labs are actually worse than Friday's.

"How does he look?"

"I haven't seen him. I don't work the floor. I'm the supervisor."

She attempts to call the floor nurse. Five minutes pass. The nurse cannot be located.

"The resident may have an infection," the nursing supervisor tells me. She has antibiotics for sensitivities (per the lab report) but cannot pronounce them.

By now, I am worried. I tell her to send the resident to the hospital.

8:23 p.m.—I receive a call regarding a simple fall. The nurse who reports the incident used to work at Fern Oakes. She has heard that the state inspectors are doing a survey there now.

"Those people [the administrative staff] will do anything to save their skin," she tells me. When I was working there, someone nabbed all my notes out of the charts. "Can you believe it?"

I am inclined to trust her.

8:35 p.m.—A nurse calls to report a skin tear to a patient when she transferred him from a bed to a chair.

9:20 p.m.—A resident has increased urinary incontinence. I order a urine culture.

9:50 p.m.—A supervisor reports labs from yesterday.

10:00 p.m.—A call comes in regarding a resident; no further information is left. I call back several times. I let the phone ring and ring. I wonder how I would feel if I were a family member calling the facility about a loved one.

10:30 p.m.—Thirty minutes have gone by with no calls. I try to sleep.

11:15 p.m.—A resident at Fern Oakes demands to be sent to the hospital. She believes that she has an infection, as she feels hot. She has just returned to the facility after using a pass to go to a bar for karaoke night. "If you don't send me to the hospital," she threatens the staff, "I'll dial 911 myself." I agree to let her go.

Monday Morning

12:55 a.m.—A resident states that she does not feel good and wants the doctor called. "There's no change in her," the nurse tells me. "Her kids are out of town, and she's probably just feeling lonely."

12:57 a.m.—A nurse calls in labs from a week ago. He is not sure if they were reported earlier.

2:05 a.m.—A new admission arrived from the hospital yesterday afternoon. Had I been called to verify his admission orders? I had not.

2:55 a.m.—A call comes in with no message left. When I call back, no one answers the phone. I fall asleep.

4:00 a.m.—An emergency room physician has just examined the resident at Fern Oakes, who asked to be sent to the hospital. He is quite annoyed. "Why have you sent her here? Her main problem seems to be alcohol intoxication."

I briefly explain the situation and thank him for his help.

4:22 a.m.—A resident wants to talk to me about sleep medicine. I guess it is not working.

6:01 a.m.—I listen to a message about a resident who is in more pain. The phone number left is wrong. I look up the number of the facility in the phone book.

6:27 a.m.—A diabetic has an increased blood sugar. I give him additional medication.

6:35 a.m.—I leave the house. Although I will remain on call until 8:00 a.m., I need to start my rounds. On the way, I call my mother. I neglected her yesterday. I had too many calls.

All told, I logged in seventy-two calls, a fairly typical number for one Sunday-to-Monday period.

16

The Way We Care Now

On Tuesday, I wake early. It is about five a.m. Downstairs I move about the quiet house alone. The rest of the family is still asleep upstairs. I check the fax machine (My office is right off the kitchen.) Twenty pages have arrived overnight. I scan them quickly for urgent information and then turn on the computer. The morning's e-mail includes an ad. Victoria's Secret is having a sale. I save this message as a little treat for later tonight, when I will have time to browse the electronic catalog. Shira, my eldest daughter at fourteen, has e-mailed a joke. I read the cute punch line and grin. Then I open my EMR (electronic medical record system) to print the names of the patients I will see today. While the list is printing, I make coffee and the kids' lunches. I check to see that their backpacks and other essentials are hanging where they should be in the front hall, easy to grab as each of them races out the front door later this morning. The printer stops. I organize my file and begin to respond to my faxes. Online, I check my bank account. Has Medicaid paid me yet? No, not surprisingly. Medicaid is notorious for low compensation and long waits for reimbursement. The wait for payment of some of my bills has been more than two years. Still, I would not refuse Medicaid residents, though many physicians understandably do.

Just before six, I have ten minutes to spare. I pour coffee into a mug and allow my mind to roam, still groggy after a fitful sleep. Yet I hope that the caffeine might stimulate an idea or two as I write this final chapter. How do I sum up and finish this book? Moments later, I can only hope that my subconscious takes over the task. The hands on the kitchen clock point to six. I take one last gulp and head upstairs, where I wake Shira and go on to do fifteen minutes of exercise before I shower and dress. The new day is now officially under way. No matter how monotonous, tedious, or stressful, it will present me with its own story.

Down the hall, a melodrama arises. Shira has lost the stone from her ring. We find it. Only then she is not pleased with how her hair looks. We solve that problem also. At six-thirty, I wake up my two younger children—Jared, who is twelve, and Avishav, who just turned eight. It is time for Shira and me to leave the house.

On the way out the door, I call up the stairs to Jared: "Be sure and put on clean clothes."

I know that he is reluctant to do so. Just the other day, he told me that "men don't change their underwear." "Promise?" I say.

"Okay, okay," he grumbles.

"I'm tired, Mom," Avishav tells me, coming to stand at the top of the stairs, "and I feel like I'm going to throw up."

"Go see Dad," I tell her. Shira and I must get going.

On my way to Carter Hill Nursing Home, I drop Shira off at Willow Lake Middle School.

"Good luck today," I say to her as she hops out of the car. "I'll do my best to be there."

"That would be great, Mom," she says and slams the door. She is nervous, I can tell.

Today is the spelling bee competition. She and her dad and I have been practicing how to spell exotic and incredibly long words for weeks.

As already chronicled, I will visit residents at several facilities this morning. Between my visits, I will stop at the grocery for some fresh food for dinner, return a pair of shoes that did not fit Avishav, and drop by Shira's school for thirty minutes to see her in the spelling bee. It has taken years to achieve some sort of seamlessness between the two sides of my life. Now it seems to have happened. The professional and the personal definitely are intertwined. As I run errands, I find my thoughts return to where I left them at six o'clock this morning. What final observations can I make before I come to the end of this notebook?

It is easy to see that the numbers of elderly and chronically ill people have risen over the last few decades. Whether their greater longevity represents a positive change in how we care now is harder to tell. Do the ill and the elderly enjoy more peace and comfort than their counterparts did in the shorter lives they led in the past?

Again, it is hard, if not impossible, to say. Caring for the elderly and the ill is hardly novel or new. Science may have improved the ways that we deliver medications to ease pain, but interestingly the main ingredients have been available since before the B.C. era—morphine and alcohol.

Can we at least claim to do a better job of providing long-term care, because of the institutional management systems that we have put into place in the last forty years? I would tend to say no, though we have become good at management.

Management systems took root after the practice of medicine left home. As late as the 1960s, physicians often operated out of offices literally attached to the sides of their own houses. Nursing homes were not corporations. Typically, they were mom-and-pop operations. Many of the caregivers who worked in such homes also lived on-site (again, the norm until the 1960s). In the forty-odd years since, we have come to opt for professional care as opposed to care offered at home. Choosing that option has grown exponentially as women entered the workforce, and families needed to pay nannies, day care centers, and long-term care facilities to provide care from the cradle to the grave.

With so many of us entering the public domain for care, institutional standards necessarily have had to be set. To protect the elderly and the ill from their own vulnerability, we have developed laws and regulations and a new professional group to monitor the institutions where we house such people. A huge and profitable industry of inspection has grown up to find flaws and breakdowns in models of care, both in the plans and the teams that execute them. The result is a system of care so intricate that it can rarely be implemented properly, despite the sophisticated strides made in management.

Unfortunately, the outcome almost always appears negative, regardless of proper care. Families count on professionals to care for their old and ill relatives, only to feel let down when their loved ones die. When that happens, can we say that management has failed? Do we have someone to blame? Of course. The doctor can be blamed for medical malpractice. Politicians can be blamed for inadequacies in the insurance industry. Perhaps even hospice can be blamed for not urging an exit from terminal care and a search for a miracle cure.

In the afternoon, I am lucky. My medical rounds go smoothly, and the crosstown traffic happen to be light. I manage to slip into the darkened auditorium of Shira's middle school just before one o'clock. The spelling bee semifinalists will vie on stage, adding a touch of theater to the event. At least I feel excited as the curtain parts, and the lights come up to reveal the thirty contestants. Vastly outnumbered by the children on stage, the audience cannot offer much of a welcoming round of applause. We consist of three women and two men, each of whom I recognize as parents and neighbors. Where is everyone else? I wonder. In our small but affluent community, many women do not work outside the home.

Several rows ahead of me, the two other mothers in the audience do not applaud at all, engrossed as they are in whispered conversation. Neither one of them turns toward the stage, where their sons will soon spell "onomatopoeia" and "portulaca," respectively and correctly.

What must their boys think?

They are used to being ignored, probably.

Of the two women, I know Joe Holliday's mom—tall, slender Esther—a bit better than I know Eric Fleischer's mom—plump and rosy Alison. Just this past winter, Esther sent her nanny to hear Joe sing in the holiday choral concert. She was too busy to come herself, as she was the chair of a gala fundraiser for the local children's home.

A bit of irony there, I think. How much time will Joe spend with his mom when she is old, I wonder.

Given my profession, I tend to speculate along these lines.

Will he care for her at home?

Or, when the time comes, will Joe follow his mom's example and opt out of her care because he is too busy, as he runs, say, a lab devoted to finding a cure for Alzheimer's disease?

Will even irony be passed like a torch from mother to son?

Here and now, in the spelling competition, Joe is beginning to leave many of the other kids behind. Obviously, he is a bright boy. Perhaps, he will be smart enough to see that institutionalized systems of care should never be mistaken for caring.

❧

A major goal of long-term care facilities is for professional care teams to function as much like families as possible. Yet the goal is elusive. If ten years of geriatrics have convinced me of anything, it is that the elderly and the ill are better off when their actual families do not surrender to the institution but remain closely involved in their elders' lives. In families where parents have had an active and loving hand in raising their children, the role reversal—where children take an active part in caring for their elders—usually comes naturally. Such families are fortunate enough to have a solid foundation to carry out what I see as an ethical system of long-term care.

As we have seen, active family participation in geriatric care is not without its shortcomings and counterproductive consequences. Families who deny the physical limitations of their relatives, or who cast a vote of no confidence in the medical and health care professions, can make the aging and dying process a miserable one for all concerned. Even so, the patients themselves are almost always better off—precisely because their families take an interest in them.

A tendency to leave most decisions to the professional care team remains the preferred option among families who are unsettled and dysfunctional. Whether they feel desperate or are simply attracted by expediency, such families tend to turn quickly to long-term care facilities to manage their relatives' care. Perhaps because there is such a need to believe it, the myth persists that the professional knows "best," even though to pay a caretaker does not guarantee excellence and, in fact, the average staff member in long-term care has but a few weeks of training, is often new on the job, and thus has no more than a passing acquaintance with residents.

Correspondingly, the more control (responsibility) the family gives up, the less say it has in the care of its elderly and ill members. With a loss of responsibility, inevitably occurs a loss of autonomy. In fact, long-term care facilities may subtly encourage families to step aside so as to gain more control of the caretaking process. The alternative is not attractive to facilities, which must be run much like any other business. The active involvement of families at the nursing home can indeed present headaches. Beyond that, were a resident to go home, a bed would be empty, the facility census would be down, and the result would be lower profits. Perhaps the return home would be bad for the scientific model too (no one to treat) and bad for social solutions. (A public domain in which to age and die would not be needed quite so much.)

Families who, for whatever reason, do not maintain an active involvement paradoxically become less and less satisfied with the systems to which they have relinquished control. Passivity and distrust build. Many families seem to be afraid that, if they voice their dissatisfaction to the staff directly, they will invite some form of retaliation, to the detriment of their elders. Instead, they let their dissatisfaction fester. Sometimes they take their cumulative displeasure to an attorney on whom, for another fee, they unburden themselves. Naturally such an approach to problem solving will lead to lawsuits.

Long-term care facilities respond to complaints and lawsuits by taking more and more precautions to protect themselves. They end up ever more proactive and defensive in an effort to be "faultless" (on paper at least). Families lose even more autonomy—and trust—as they confront an administrative fortress. The main consequence of this unfortunate cycle is the erosion of quality care, as energy and resources are marshaled for defensive purposes. Another casualty is medicine itself, which has gone from being a caring and spiritual profession to a service profession. The personal rapport and trust that used to be built as part of a physician-patient relationship have deteriorated, too. Medicine is falsely viewed as an exact science in which uncertainties and risks are subject to litigation. The truth is medicine is an art based on science.

The spelling bee is nearly over, and I am literally on the edge of my seat. The thirty semifinalists have dwindled down to three—Joe, Eric, and Shira. With a letter-perfect rendition of the word "Inuktitut," my daughter beats out Eric and takes second place behind Joe, who wins the bee by spelling "limitrophe" correctly with a middle "i," whereas Shira spells it incorrectly with a middle "a." I clap wildly and manage to reach out and give my daughter's shoulder a squeeze as she and her classmates file out of the auditorium, and we in the tiny audience begin to leave.

As I move up the aisle, I feel a hand on my elbow and turn to see Joe's mom, Esther Holliday.

"Congratulations," I say.

"Thanks," she says. "It did come off beautifully, didn't it?"

"You have a very bright son."

For a moment she looks startled, and then flashes me a smile. "Oh, right, of course I do. Thanks very much. Actually, though, I was thinking of the gala. You and Abe attended, I remember."

"Yes, it was great," I agree, as I try to be gracious and move toward the parking lot as quickly as possible.

"Well, it was my pleasure," Esther continues, blocking my way up the aisle, "—but a lot of work."

"I'm sure." I look at my watch.

"Anyway, Gilah. We're looking for volunteers for the school carnival in June. Would you be willing? It won't take much time. Nothing like the gala."

I am tempted to say that we are going to be out of town. I think again. Maybe I should volunteer? Finally, I say what I really want to say.

"Sorry, Esther. I'm really overextended at the moment."

"How about a mere thirty minutes to run a booth?"

"I really can't," I say and gently move around her to continue toward the exit. Halfway up the aisle, I turn back to face her. "Besides, I'd only be robbing Peter to pay Paul."

Esther's quizzical look tells me that she has no idea what I mean: My own family and my patients come first. To volunteer at school, I would have to cut into their time. This risk is not one I'm prepared to take, even for the best of causes. Or, should I say, my family and my patients are my causes? I truly am already overextended and have to choose my priorities carefully. My guarded stance reminds of just how risk-averse my profession has come to be.

To withstand legal and regulatory challenges, nursing homes must remain vigilant. Their first line of defense is to screen their prospective residents. Obviously, some prospects are more desirable than others. The compliant individual who has undergone an elective hip replacement and has good insurance is certainly less of a business risk than, say, the homeless elder who has wounds that need constant treatment but no insurance coverage at all. Such are the calculations that encourage admissions decisions that play it safe.

Will it soon become too risky to maintain residents in long-term-care facilities? The question may sound absurd, but already the insurance industry has decided to discourage physicians from working in such institutions because of the legal risks. Our mechanized and regulated form of caring can make life itself seem too risky to live. I think again of the poem that one of my first patients thrust at me, just as I was starting out as a nursing home doctor ten years ago.

I am an intruder, observer, spectator, bystander, and witness.
I work here but do not live here.
I am employed by the sky that "they" say is blue, yet I don't see it as blue.
The boss is purple. The clouds are green.
The boss is not God but rules us fiercer than God would—
This leader has no morals.
I know more than "you" know,
Yet I am ostracized. You have a promotion.
I am sad yet content,
I am lonely and sexy,
But I am empowered.
My wishes have been fulfilled.
I have succeeded,
But I am hopeless.
I can no longer dream.
My fears have never materialized.
I have been lucky,
But I am still afraid.
You are me but afraid of the risk.
You are managed.

I return again to the same questions I jotted down in response: Have we come to manage so much that we would manage (and muzzle) God, too, if we could? Is hedging against loss, misfortune, or injury—as we do in long-term care—more important than complying with absolute principles of ethics, such as compassion and humility? What drives us to expend our energies on combating the unchangeable—meaning aging and death—yet retracting when we should reach out to comfort and to offer simple, human companionship? Does documentation shield us not only from lawsuits but also from honest acknowledgment of what it is to age and to die?

After the bee, I stop by my home office. My home is my office, and my office is my home. I like it this way, just as I like to think of myself as a modern woman practicing old-fashioned medicine. Fifty faxes await. I respond to them, update my files on the patients I saw this morning, and print out a ream of medical records. I get the mail and sort it. In the kitchen I make several phone calls as I start dinner and make a snack for the kids to eat after school. Then it is time to go pick them up. On the way out the door, I grab a book in case I get to the elementary school well before the bell rings. These days I am reading *The Wine Bible*, as my husband, Abe, has become interested in learning about the different growers and their vintages. All wine still tastes about the same to me. Unlike Abe, I have not paid much attention to the details. I did not recall, for example, that there was a dry season in Bordeaux in 1977 when he mentioned the fact the other night. I would find a small glass of wine a nice way to relax even if Bordeaux were part of Oregon. Today before I walk across the street to pick up my two youngest, I make a resolution. I will read *The Wine Bible* for twenty minutes tomorrow and impress Abe. Do I really need to impress someone I have lived with for twenty-two years? I think so.

Many parents use the car line, but I like to walk into the building and look at the artwork and projects on display. On days like this one when I arrive before three, I can spot my two kids out on the playground. Avishav smiles brightly when she sees me and waves. My son, Jared, tries to ignore me, but sometimes I have caught him out in a smile also.

As I look out across the asphalt filled with vibrant young children, the question pops into my head: When do we realize our mortality?

Surely not often in sunny moments like these.

It is often said that we make the realization when we see a relative or a friend die.

In my experience, the recognition does not occur until we experience physical or mental failure personally. We come to recognize our own mortality from within ourselves.

When we cannot walk, or see, or hear as well as we used to do.

When we can no longer work or play the way we once did—when even perseverance will not permit us to succeed.

That is when we recognize our mortality.

In the meantime, could it be that our fear of mortality has forced us to develop a care plan for death but not an acceptance of death? Has the artificial complexity of such a plan, which we have constructed, served to hide our basic fears and disguise our mortality?

The idea that aging and death can be managed implies that aging and death can be "solved." If we just play our cards right, we can waylay the inevitable more or less indefinitely.

We pile into the car, and for the third time today I drive over to the middle school, where we will pick up Shira.

"How did your day go? I ask my two youngest.

"Fine," they each say as usual.

The difference is that, at eight, Avishav sounds carefree, whereas, at twelve, Jared sounds sullen and suspicious. "Why do you ask?" is how he often responds to my ordinary, everyday questions these days.

"Shira did well in the spelling bee," I tell them. "No, don't turn on the radio yet," I add as Jared reaches for the dial. "It's shift change in the nursing homes. I have five pages to answer."

From the back seat, Avishav groans. "Aw, Mom. You always do that. It's not fair. We want to listen to music."

"Live with it," Jared tells her. Today he plays mature older brother, which is not always the case.

There have been days when I had to stop the car and calm them down. I cannot permit them to complain, as I would prefer. I have nurses on the phone asking me questions. Today, however, Avishav goes along with her brother's advice to be stoic. The two of them munch on the snacks I have brought along while I drive more or less with my elbows—phone in one hand, pager in the other. Stopped at a traffic light for a second, I even try to write some of the information that I am receiving down on a slip of paper. The light turns green, and I run up over the curb a bit. My son screams as his drink spills on his designer jeans and basketball jersey. Avishav laughs. "It's roller coaster time!" Actually, I have never gotten into an auto accident.

Ten minutes later, I finish my last call with the staff at Sweet Penny Tree. "Okay. You can turn on the radio now."

Jared tunes into a station that plays rap. Surprising myself, I have come to tolerate and even to like rap. Yet already from the back seat, Avishav is groaning again, "I hate this song! Make him change the station, Mom." Somehow we always get into a fight over what to play on the radio, despite much common ground.

We make it to the middle school without mishap and wait while Shira says goodbye to her friends and heads down the steep set of stairs in the pair of high heels she wore today. My feet hurt with her, but somehow she manages to maneuver gracefully and without falling. I am proud. As she climbs into the car, all three of us congratulate her on her performance in the "bee."

She kisses me and thanks me for coming as she settles in next to Avishav, who slaps her a "high-five."

As we drive away from her school, Shira is only half-joking when she asks, "So why didn't you dress like the other mothers today, Mom? You know the drill, don't you? You're supposed to wear beige slacks and a Ralph Lauren shirt."

She lets out a hoot of derision. Avishav joins in, although she does not quite understand why Shira is poking fun of me.

"Who cares about clothes, anyway," Jared tries to defend me from Shira.

"Mom does," Shira says.

"Yeah, I'm a fashion slave," I joke to my son.

I've been told that I've never been seen wearing the same thing twice—not entirely true. Today I wear a leather skirt and matching jacket in a soft shade of brown that complements my jade jewelry.

"Sheesh," is all that Jared has to say.

Then Shira decides to give me a break. "You may not dress like everyone else, but at least you're a well-known doctor. Even snobs respect you."

It is difficult, apparently, to write off someone whose skills may come in handy someday. Though I say nothing to Shira, I cannot say that I am eager to offer my services to our wealthy neighbors. I have done so enough to know that I must curb my bias and take each case individually.

As a whole, I have found the rich to be demanding—quick to find fault and assign blame, no matter how much time and attention they receive from me and facility staff. They also tend to be manipulative in (what they seem to think) is a sophisticated way, say, by dropping a hint that they are friends with the chairman of the board of the facility, or that their next-door neighbor is a geriatrician also, or even that their son is a lawyer who specializes in medical malpractice. Interestingly, such folk tend not to care much for me, either. I like to treat everyone as important and special, not just the so-called VIPs. Fortunately, I am able to decline patients and their families with whom I do not feel compatible. I am paid about the same, regardless of a patient's socioeconomic status. (Insurance has largely fixed and standardized my compensation.)

The practice of picking and choosing patients based, for example, on the degree of difficulty or insurance risk, is not uncommon in an age when we all fear legal repercussions. My rule for taking on a patient is actually quite simple. I will accept any resident as long as they accept me. In my many years of practice, I have never "fired" a resident. On occasion, I have been fired by a family (fairly rare). Usually, it has been a relief. However, I cannot say that I did not take it somewhat personally. As a practitioner, my low moments have come when I have been manipulated or lied to by family or care team members for their own gain. Unfortunately, such behavior is not uncommon. I have adjusted to such experiences somewhat and forget about them more quickly than I used to do. My most triumphant moments have occurred when people have told me how I influenced their lives in a positive manner. Often, what they recall is something that I barely remember doing.

Shira's remark about my dressing differently than the other mothers at the spelling bee this afternoon reminds me that I do not exactly blend into the crowd. In our small city, I do not belong to either of what I find to be distressingly polarized "cliques"—the career moms on one side and the stay-at-home moms on the other.

I am employed, yet I take care of my kids—the career moms rely on professional childcare. They hire nannies and other employees and rarely are seen at school. I doubt that they are seen much by their children, either.

I take care of my kids—yet I am employed. The stay-at-home moms cannot relate—we keep different hours—and perhaps different priorities. Even among these women, the hiring of nannies is not uncommon. In an era of professional caregiving, I have gone through medical school, residency, and entered medical practice with three young children, all of whom I gave birth to at home. I have never hired a nanny or sent a young child to day care. We have never used a babysitter outside the family (except for a few hours on an occasional weekend night), and I work full-time.

When I was a medical student and resident and needed to be gone from home, sometimes up to forty-eight hours at a time, I brought along with me a plastic cooler with ice elements and pumped and saved breast milk. Abe came and picked up the milk every twelve hours or so to feed to my babies in bottles. In this way, Shira and Jared were each breast-fed for a year. Avishav was luckier—no bottled breast milk for her ever. Five days after her birth, I returned to work with my newest baby in tow.

As parents, my husband and I require our children to study and get good grades. We encourage them to maintain a circle of friends. We do not, however, require them to play soccer, join the scouts, or take piano lessons. Soccer is a game, not a religion. Our kids are well adjusted and happy. If they have problems, the main one is not spending enough time with their friends, who are involved in many extracurricular activities. Unfortunately, it is not unusual to have to schedule a play date with a preschooler a month in advance.

Does this pattern of family devotion mean that I will succeed in taking care of my parents in old age? Of course not. The best of intentions offer no guarantees. Does living by these lights mean that my own kids will take good care of me when I am old? I have no way of knowing, nor do I believe in a simple "quid pro quo." Virtue, I have found is indeed its own reward.

Do my patients suffer from my dedication to my family? If anything, I think that they benefit. The same habits of care developed at home are carried over to the workplace and into my care of them. My method of dealing with residents and their own families is largely successful because I follow a few basic rules:

- Respond promptly. Once a family finds that I am readily accessible, they "bother" me less. The greatest fear of residents (or family members) is to be left alone when they wish most to consult with their doctor. When I first meet families, I always leave them with ways to get in touch with me (usually a business card) whether they ask for it or not.
- Be courteous. It is my job to talk to residents and their families in a respectful manner, even if they do not appear to respect me. Good treatment may eventually rub off.
- Urge individual decisions. When several options are available to treat a particular problem, I urge the family to choose the course of action that they will be most able to live with.
- Be nonjudgmental. I do, however, express personal opinions when I feel that they will really make a difference.
- Be available but set limits. One person should serve as a family's point of contact.
- Notify of absences. Before I go away on vacation, and before I take a day or two off, I make certain that residents and families know when I will be gone and when I will return. I stress that I have backup for emergencies but not for small talk.

My work at each nursing facility actually constitutes several jobs. First, I care for the medical needs of the residents and respond to the needs and requests of their families. Second, but no less important, I become part of the care team. My love for human psychology takes root here, as I can be a member of fifteen to twenty care teams at a time.

My biggest challenge in coming to a new facility is to blend in with the care team. For that reason, I spend at least half of my time with the team members. If I succeed in bonding with them, my life will be easier, and my residents will benefit in terms of their care. The above rules apply to my dealings with each facility care team, with one addition:

- Be on guard. As a member of a nursing home care team, no matter how good and devoted I am, I can be replaced in a "New York Minute."

I love what I do and hope not to be asked to leave. Still, physicians seem to be as risky as patients in the geriatric—or dying—field. Perhaps someone will see me as a risk or the facility will undergo a "culture change." I can be replaced, but not, I believe, by a doctor more dedicated than I am to the patient, and not by one more flexible with the family, or more respectful of the staff's autonomy.

৵

On Monday afternoons the kids and I stop at Starbucks on the way home from school, and today is no exception. We are regulars, so our order is prepared practically before we enter the shop. As we head to a table, Avishav spies a new breed of spider on the floor (She is a bug collector).

"Stop that," Shira hisses.

"What's the matter?" Avishav and I look up at her. Each of us holds a paper cup in pursuit of the spider.

She rolls her eyes at us. "Thanks a lot. I can never come back here anymore."

Our behavior has embarrassed her, especially since the new "espresso dude" is cute.

Luckily, we behave better after the spider is secured: Three children drink their cappuccinos while Mom spends most of her time on the phone. On the way out, the espresso maker smiles at us. I am not sure if it is because he thinks Shira is cute, also, or because we are good tippers.

At four o'clock, we arrive home. The kids have a half-hour of free, or "unwind" time. Then homework is started. Shira supervises the younger ones. In the interim, I continue to answer calls and faxes and enter into my EMR the new residents that I have seen today. At five-thirty, Shira helps me with dinner. Tonight we have bean chili. Avishav is not pleased with her meal, so I make some instant macaroni and cheese. Interestingly, I have seen families demand that a nursing home facility provide an alternate diet—immediately—for their parent. Would they be as quick to give their child an alternate meal after a hard day's work? I hope so.

At six thirty, the children finish eating. I continue to respond to faxes and a few calls. By seven, however, life calms down considerably.

My pages will now go to the physician on call for the night. I am free until eight tomorrow morning. Of course, the fax machine still prints. I answer when I feel it is appropriate.

On occasion, I will get a call at home, as I do tonight. It is the nursing supervisor at Sweet Penny Lane. She is relaying a message from the woman who called me over the weekend to demand that I order tests for her mother, based on what she learned on the Internet.

Tonight when I return her call, she sounds apologetic and anxious to seek advice.

"Is Mom dying—does she need hospice?"

I offer my thoughts. Obviously, the woman cares enormously for her mother and dreads the thought of her death.

The younger kids have gone downstairs to finish their homework. Shira stays upstairs with me. We play some music. I pour a glass of wine, and we go out to my porch, where Shira tells me about her life. As I listen, I sign my name to all of the orders I have given by telephone throughout the day. Even my teenager's stories cannot make this task more interesting.

At seven-thirty, I go downstairs to help Avishav with her five-hundred-piece jigsaw puzzle in progress. I feel guilty that I do not spend enough time with her and offer her five more minutes. She declines and wants to play on the GameCube with her brother.

"Don't worry, Mom," she reassures me. "We can do more tomorrow." I guess that I am not so important after all.

By nine o'clock, bath time is over, and I have said goodnight to my children. I settle in at my computer and browse the Victoria's Secret sale. I think I need a new skirt. I place an order and then sit down to bean chili and a cabernet sauvignon with my husband. We watch *Real Time with Bill Maher* and an old episode of *Sex in the City*. Drowsy but content, I have but one last note to add to this book.

What if more families were to resume direct care of their members? Were the family to retake more of its former control, the business of long-term care would not wither away. There might be less need for institutional care, but the need itself would not disappear. Science, insurance, and hospice would remain in demand as quite useful, when selected on á la carte basis to fulfill particular family needs and to complement their varying structures. If used properly, the marketable systems related to long-term care could complete and enhance the ethical model, yet not take strong root and supplant the family.

On its face, such a proposal is not particularly realistic, I suppose. As caretakers of our families, we have less and less experience as we evolve as a society. Yet care for another human being cannot really be bought. If the family recedes, so does personal connection and concern.

I doze off on the sofa and dream of the spelling bee earlier in the day.

Without a moment's hesitation, Joe Holliday spells "sortilege" correctly and then points his finger at me, out in the audience. "It's her fault," he shouts

"I put Mom in that nursing home for the best of care. Now something's wrong with her, and it's her fault."

I awake with a start but am not surprised. Joe is a likely candidate to step back from direct involvement in the terminal care of his distant and preoccupied mother. All the same, he is enough of a perfectionist to blame the doctor for whatever ails her. Oh well. Maybe Eric Fleischman will behave better, I think, trying to cheer myself up.

www.ingramcontent.com/pod-product-compliance
Lightning Source LLC
Chambersburg PA
CBHW070420290526
45791CB00005B/1766

* 9 7 8 1 4 1 9 6 7 3 2 5 2 *